AF334889

Recent Results
in Cancer Research

151

Managing Editors
P.M. Schlag, Berlin · H.-J. Senn, St. Gallen

Associate Editors
V. Diehl, Cologne · D.M. Parkin, Lyon
M.F. Rajewsky, Essen · R. Rubens, London
M. Wannenmacher, Heidelberg

Founding Editor
P. Rentchnik, Geneva

Springer

*Berlin
Heidelberg
New York
Barcelona
Hong Kong
London
Milan
Paris
Singapore
Tokyo*

H.-J. Senn   A. Costa   V.C. Jordan   (Eds.)

Chemoprevention of Cancer

A Clinical Update

With 19 Figures and 18 Tables

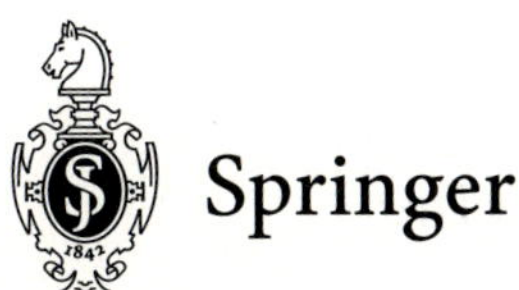

Springer

Prof. Dr. med. Hans-Jörg Senn
Center for Tumordetection and Prevention
Rorschacherstrasse 150
CH-9006 St. Gallen

Dr. Alberto Costa, M.D.
European Institute of Oncology
Via Ripamonti
I-20141 Milan

Prof. M.D., Ph.D. V.Craig Jordan
Robert H. Lurie Cancer Center
Breast Cancer Research Program
Olson Pavilion, Northwest-University Medical School
503 E. Chicago Ave.
Chicago, IL 60611, USA

ISBN 3-540-64710-4 Springer-Verlag Berlin Heidelberg New York
ISSN 0080-0015

Library of Congress Cataloging-in-Publication Data
Chemoprevention of cancer: a clinical update / H.-J. Senn, A. Costa, C. Jordan. p.cm. – (Recent results in cancer research, ISSN 0080-0015; 151) Contains the lectures of the 2nd Annual Conference of the International Society of Cancer Chemoprevention held Aug. 1997 in St. Gallen, Switzerland. Includes bibliographical references and index. ISBN 3-540-64710-4 (hardcover: alk. paper) 1. Cancer – Chemoprevention – Congresses. I. Senn, Hansjörg. II. Costa, A. (Alberto) III. Jordan, Craig. IV: International Society of Cancer Chemoprevention. Conference. (2nd: 1997: Saint Gallen, Switzerland) V. Series. [DNLM: 1. Neoplasms – prevention & control congresses. 2. Chemoprevention congresses. W1RE106P v. 151 1998]. RC261.R35 vol. 151 [RC268.15] 616.99′4 s – dc21 [616.99′4052] DNLM/DLC for Library of Congress.

Production: PRO EDIT GmbH, D-69126 Heidelberg
Typesetting: K+V Fotosatz GmbH, D-64743 Beerfelden

SPIN 10658643   19/3133-5 4 3 2 1 0 – Printed on acid-free paper

Preface

Pharmacologic interventions to prevent the evolution of human cancers are still in its infancy, although a good number of – mostly controlled – clinical studies have been performed in the past two decades. However, regarding the partially stagnating therapeutic results of major epithelial cancer types such as breast-, lung-, colon- and ENT-cancer types, the problem of interference with the evolution of disease at a preclinical level is an intriguing one, and the field seems to develop into one of the fastest growing domaines of modern oncology. This process is facilitated by the developments of molecular onco-genetics and the gowing existence of family cancer units, allowing to better identify and inform respective high risk groups, thus enabling researchers and clinicians to more realistically target their chemopreventive efforts to the true populations at risk.

On this changing background, the newly formed International Society of Cancer Chemoprevention (ISCaC) together with the Swiss Cancer League and the Interdisciplinary Oncology Center of St. Gallen/Switzerland organized an international Symposium in September 1997, inviting basic researchers, epidemiologists and clinical oncologists of related disciplines to discuss pertinent issues of experimental and clinical chemo- and bio-prevention in a scientific workshop. This was one of the first efforts to units experts of major groups and centers worldwide in this highly fascinating and thought-provoking field of chemoprevention, as the meeting was very broad in its table of content, ranging form smoking, genetics and lung cancer to targets and markers for cancer prevention and the identification of meaningful high risk groups for cancer chemoprevention into the still cumbersome efforts of clinical studies in the field.

It is this last domaine, where drawbacks and contradictory results have been encountered in the recent past. Although there have been more than 60 more or less randomized trials of some chemopreventive efforts reported, only a small fraction of those could be termed as so-called definitive trials, involving different endpoints [1]. A remarkable survey is presented by Scott Lippman et al. in a recent issue of the Journal of the National Cancer Institute [2]. Unfortunately, only very few trials such as the – prematurely closed – breast cancer prevention trial with tamoxifen of the NSABP have reported "positive" results, and even these have been greatly challenged and critisized at an international level! Unfortunately, the breast cancer prevention trials were not yet "ready" for presentation and citation in fall of 1997, and therefore could not be included in this presented meeting report.

It is therefore imperative, that intensified research at the basic as well as clinical level and the dialogue between researchers and clinicians are continuing regularly in chemoprevention, in order to make realistic steps forwards in this fascinating field of oncology of the future. The development of valid surrogate end-points and biomarkers to indicate interventional drug activity, along with realistic risk models, would greatly enhance the development and conduct of shorter and less expensive chemopreventive studies [2].

References

1. Sporn MB, Lippman SM (1997) Chemoprevention of cancer. In: Holland JF, Frei E, Bast RC jr., Kufe DW, Morton DL, Weichselbaum RR (eds) Cancer Medicine, 4th Edition, Baltimore, Williams & Wilkins, p 495–508
2. Lippman SM, Lee J, Sabichi AL (1998) Cancer Chemoprevention: Progress and Promise. J Nat Cancer Inst 90:1514–1528

St. Gallen, in December 1998   *Hans-Jörg Senn*

Contents

IV. Clinical Cancer Chemoprevention

List of Contributors[*]

Amos, C. I.[3]
Bagnasco, M.[29]
Bennicelli, C.[29]
Bonithon-Kopp, C.[122]
De Flora, S.[29]
De Vries, N.[13]
Faivre, J.[122]
Fürstenberger, G.[45]
Jordan, V. C.[96]
Marks, F.[45]

Meyskens, F. L.[113]
Morrow, M.[85]
Müller-Decker, K.[45]
Pasterino, U.[13]
Scott, R. J.[71]
Sobol, H. H.[71]
Spitz, M. R.[3]
Van Zandwijk, N.[13]
Wu, X.[3]

---

[*] The address of the principal author is given on the first page of each contribution.
[1] Page on which contribution begins.

I. Smoking, Genetics and Cancer

Is There a Genetic Basis for Lung Cancer Susceptibility?

C. I. Amos, W. Xu, and M. R. Spitz

Department of Epidemiology, University of Texas M. D. Anderson Cancer Center, 1515 Holcombe Blvd., Box 189, Houston, TX 77030, USA

Abstract

The major risk factor for lung cancer is exposure to tobacco smoke. Exposure to radon, heavy metals used in smelting, and asbestos also greatly increase risks for lung cancer. However, only about 11% of tobacco smokers ultimately develop lung cancer, suggesting that genetic factors may influence the risk for lung cancer among those who are exposed to carcinogens. Further support for this hypothesis is provided by several epidemiological studies and also from molecular epidemiological studies. Epidemiological studies show approximately 14-fold increased risks for lung cancer among average tobacco smokers and approximately 2.5-fold increased risks attributable to a family history of lung cancer after controlling for tobacco smoke. Segregation analyses suggest that a rare autosomal dominant gene may explain susceptibility to early-onset lung cancer, but these results explain a minority of lung cancer cases, which include a familiy history. Therefore, more common genetic variants or polymorphisms are hypothesized to affect lung cancer risk. Environmental carcinogenesis resulting from tobacco smoke exposure is a complex process that can involve activation of procarcinogens that lead to adduct formation and subsequent failure of DNA repair, which should normally remove these adducts. Studies comparing DNA repair capacity among newly diagnosed lung cancer patients and age-matched controls indicate significant differences between the two groups. On culturing with bleomycin lymphocytes from lung cancer patients and age- and ethnicity-matched controls, the lymphocytes from lung cancer cases have been consistently observed to show higher levels of chromatid breaks than the control lymphocytes. A similar assay has been developed using benzo-[a]pyrene diol-epoxide (BPDE), a reactive substrate that is derived by in vitro processes from benzo[a]pyrene, a major carcinogen in tobacco smoke. Results from this assay show an even more significantly higher level of damaged chromatids in lung cancer patients than in controls. Poor DNA repair is independent of tobacco smoking status. The cellular processes involved in DNA repair of bleomycin and BPDE have not yet been fully elaborated. However, the consistency of findings with these two carcinogens indi-

Recent Results in Cancer Research, Vol. 151
Senn/Costa/Jordan (Eds.): Chemoprevention of Cancer
© Springer-Verlag Berlin · Heidelberg 1999

cates that DNA repair capacity influences risk for lung cancer among individuals.

Introduction

The major determinant of lung cancer susceptibility in humas is exposure to carcinogenic compounds in common environmental pollutants, including tobacco smoke, asbestos, aromatic hydrocarbons commonly occurring in the petrochemical industry, and metals. However, the influence of familial factors in determining lung cancer risk was well established over 30 years ago (Tokuhata and Lillienfeld 1963), and ample evidence from animal studies documents genetic effects on lung cancer susceptibility (Nebert 1991). Although the familial nature of lung cancer has long been well established, progress in characterizing and then identifiying the specific genetic factors that influence lung cancer susceptibility in humans has been slow.

Familial Aggregation Studies in Lung Cancer

One approach to characterizing genetic susceptibility for lung cancer consists of family studies of lung cancer cases. The landmark study of Tokuhata and Lillienfeld (1963) demonstrated excess lung cancer mortality among the relatives of lung cancer patients. Synergism was observed between smoking behavior and the occurrence of lung cancer in the patients' relatives. For men, environmental determinants predominated, while for women, genetic or familial factors were more important. With controls who did not smoke, as the referent group, the risks associated with smoking and familial factors were: a 4-fold increase in mortality among patients' relatives who did not smoke, a 5-fold increase in mortality among controls' relatives who smoked, and a 14-fold increase in mortality among relatives of patients who smoked. Ooi et al. (1986) confirmed these findings in a study of 337 lung cancer cases from Southern Louisiana and their spouse controls. This study yielded an odds ratio for lung cancer, after adjustment for smoking behavior and occupational exposure, of 2.4 associated with having a relative with lung cancer.

Studies of risk for cancer at other sites (Sellers et al. 1987) showed an odds ratio of 4.6 for head and neck cancers, 2.8 for skin cancers, and 2.7 for thyroid cancer. McDuffie (1991) found an 8.3-fold risk for vocal cord/esophageal cancers in males and an infinite odds ratio in females (6 cases in 1225 relatives of cases versus 0 cases in 835 relatives of controls). Risks for sites other than the lung (which had a 1.96 odds ratio in males and 1.78 odds ratio in females) were not significantly increased, but the risk ratio for pancreatic cancer in females was infinite (7 cases in relatives of cases, versus 0 cases in relatives of controls). Schwartz et al. (1996), studying nonsmoking patients with lung cancer, found an increased risk associated with family history of 7.2 among young cases (less than age 60), but no increased risk associated with family history among older nonsmoking patients.

Segregation analyses have been conducted to fit genetic models to family data. Results of analysis (Sellers et al. 1990) of the data collected by Ooi et al. (1986) were consistent with Mendelian segregation of a codominant locus affecting the age at onset for development of lung cancer, after allowing for effects from smoking behaviors. Further analysis of these data (Gauderman et al. 1997) to allow for missing data concerning smoking exposures led to the conclusion that an autosomal dominant model with a gene frequency of about 2% provided the best fit to the data. Neither recessive nor codominant models could be rejected, but nongenetic models were rejected. Carriers of disease susceptibility in this model had a 17-fold increased risk for developing lung cancer, and there was no significant evidence for statistical interaction between smoking and genetic susceptibility on the logistic (or mulitplicative) scale. Analysis of data from relatives of nonsmoking cases studied by Schwartz et al. (1996) was not consistent with effects from a single major gene (Yang et al. 1997). Instead, the results were most consistent with risk attributable to both measured and unmeasured environmental agents. Results from these studies do not provide a clear model to explain familial patterns of lung cancer. However, the models that can be fitted to family data are unable to capture effects from models more complex than simple Mendelian or polygenic inheritance unless genetic linkage data are available.

Because genetic modeling strategies may not be reliable for modeling complex diseases such as lung cancer, alternative approaches to the identification of genetic factors in the etiology of lung cancer have been sought. Genetic linkage approaches have been highly successful in the study of other rare familial cancers, such as hereditary nonpolyposis colon cancer (Aaltonen 1993) and breast cancer (Miki et al. 1994). For lung cancer, the genetic linkage approach, which requires sampling of extended families including numerous affected relatives, is difficult to implement. Relatives of affected individuals are often deceased. Tumor blocks are also often not available from affected individuals as they often would be in the case of breast or colon cancer. Although efforts are currently under way in the United States to conduct genetic linkage analysis for lung cancer, these studies require a concerted effort involving large numbers of collaborating investigators to obtain sufficient informative families. An alternative approach that can be effective in identifying more common genetic variations associated with more modest risks uses molecular epidemiological approaches.

Molecular Epidemiological Studies of Lung Cancer Susceptibility

Substantial evidence has suggested that the carcinogenic process is driven by the interaction of exogenous carcinogenic exposures and inherent genetic traits. The internal dose of carcinogens may be modulated by genetic polymorphisms in the enzymes responsible for activation and detoxification of these carcinogens. The polymorphisms on these carcinogen-metabolic enzymes have been shown to be susceptibility markers for lung cancer (Wu et al. 1997; Kawajiri et al. 1995; Nakachi et al. 1993). In addition to variation in carcinogen-metabolic enzymes, individual variability in response to environmental mutagens may be mediated by susceptibility to chromosome damage resulting from environmental exposures and by rates of DNA repair (Setlow 1978; Glickman 1980; Bohr et al. 1987; Hsu et al. 1993).

It is likely that there is considerable interindividual variation in sensitivity to environmental mutagens, i.e., some individuals may be highly resistant to mutagens and others may have a sensitivity close to those of the instability syndromes (Hsu 1983). Thus, under similar environmental exposure conditions, a person who has a slight defect in one step of DNA repair may accumulate more mutations and chromosomal aberrations than another individual with intact repair systems. Therefore, persons with defects in any step of DNA or chromosome repair could be classified as being in an at-risk category. In addition, it is possible that individuals may have variant sequences that are more susceptible to DNA damage from clastogens (Yunis et al. 1987). The balance of inherent genomic instability and DNA repair capacity along with ability to metabolize carcinogenic factors results in an individual-specific profile risk from any particular carcinogen.

Hsu and colleagues have developed a mutagen sensitivity assay based on the quantification of bleomycin-induced chromatid breaks in cultured lymphocytes to measure human susceptibility to environmental carcinogens (Hsu et al. 1989; Spitz et al. 1993, 1995; Strom et al. 1995; Hsu et al. 1991; Schantz et al. 1990). A measurement error study (Cloos et al. 1993) showed that mean interindividual variation (0.35) exceeded mean intraindividual variation (0.08). The average number of chromatid breaks per cell (b/c) needed to evaluate individual specific risk has been extensively studied (Lee et al. 1996). After evaluation of counts from 100 metaphase spreads, it was found that after the first 50 metaphases, the theoretical gain in reducing the standard error of the proportion of breaks per metaphase spread was <1% with each additional reading. The findings suggest that the conventional method of reading 50 metaphases can yield an acceptable reliability for epidemiological studies (Lee et al. 1996).

Hsu has suggested that the bleomycin lymphocyte assay indirectly measures the effectiveness of one or more DNA repair mechanisms. A correlation between DNA repair capacity and mutagen sensitivity has also been reported (Wei et al. 1996). However, Pandita and Hittelman (1995) suggested that mutagen sensitivity may also involve an inherent chromatin alteration that permits more efficient translocation of DNA damage into chromosome damage following mutagen exposure. They found increased levels of initial chromosome damage (detected by premature chromosome condensation), a reduced fast repair component, and higher residual chromosome damage in lymphoblastoid cell lines from bleomycin-hypersensitive patients with multiple primary head and neck tumors than in those from normal control patients.

Until the mechanistic basis of bleomycin sensitivity is known in more detail, however, the assay must be viewed as a measure of relative susceptibility that may represent the composite results of multiple processes. As described below, the strong and consistent associations between bleomycin sensitivity and risk of certain environmental related cancers suggest that it measures a potentially informative aspect of suceptibility to damage or of repair capacity in those tissues.

Bleomycin Sensitivity and Lung Cancer Risk

By using a molecular epidemiologic approach, we have consistently demonstrated in case-control studies that bleomycin sensitivity based on quantification of bleomycin-induced chromatid breaks in short-term cultured PBLs is a significant independent cancer risk predictor for lung cancer and upper aerodigestive tract cancers (Hsu et al. 1989, 1991; Strom et al. 1995; Wu et al. 1995; Spitz et al. 1989, 1993). In a case-control study of lung cancer with 180 cases and 270 age, sex, and ethnicity-matched controls, we found that the overall odds ratio (OR) (95% confidence interval [CL]) for bleomycin sensitivity (dichotomized at 1 break/cell) in lung cancer risk after adjusting for ethnicity and smoking status was 4.3 (2.3, 7.9) (Wu et al. 1995). The OR (95% CL) for current smokers was 2.9 (1.3, 6.5). For former smokers and never smokers, the OR (95% CL) were even higher: 4.8 (2.2, 10.5) and 8.1 (1.9, 34.3), respectively. Lighter smokers (those who smoked <1 pack per day) appeared to be at higher risk (OR = 5.7) than heavier smokers (OR = 3.2). The data were also dichotomized at 61 years of age (the median age of the cases and controls). The OR (95% CL) for mutagen sensitivity for younger patients was 7.8 (2.8, 21.5), as against 2.7 (1.2, 6.2) for older patients. These findings are consistent with the hypothesis that extremely mutagen-sensitive individuals are susceptible to cancer development at earlier ages than less sensitive individuals, even in the absence of overwhelming environmental exposures such as cigarette smoking. When the subjects were categorized into quartiles of breaks/cell values, with 0.50 break/cell as the referent category, a dose-response relationship between mutagen sensitivity and lung cancer risk was apparent.

The sensitivity profiles (mean chromatide breaks/cell) of both cases and controls were not affected by current or former smoking status or pack-year history, although the values for cases were consistently higher than those for controls (Spitz et al. 1995; Wu et al. 1995). There was no trend for increasing mutagen sensitivity with greater exposure. Furthermore, the duration of cessation was unrelated to the breaks/cell value. Tumor stage was also not predicted by the breakage score. Thus, this phenotype appears to be constitutionally expressed.

Stratified analysis showed that there was a synergistic interaction between mutagen sensitivity and current and former smoking and heavy smoking (Spitz et al. 1995). Gene-environmental interaction in lung cancer risk is suggested. We found a synergistic interaction between mutagen sensitivity and *CYP2E1* c1/c1 genotype in lung cancer risk (Wu et al. 1997). This phenomenon might be due in part to an increase in tobacco *N*-nitrosamine activation by *CYP2E1* to form alkyl intermediates. This induction could play a key role in smoking-related cancer.

Although consistently elevated in patients with head and neck, colon, and lung cancers, bleomycin sensitivity of patients with tumors of the breast or central nervous system did not differ from control values (Hsu et al. 1989). It has been hypothesized that the role of bleomycin sensitivity in cancer susceptibility is most pronounced at sites that are directly and chronically exposed to environmental carcinogens (Hsu et al. 1989). Thus, these data support the notion that mutagen sensitivity can be a marker for environment-related cancer susceptibility.

BPDE (Benzo[*a*]pyrene Diol Epoxide) Sensitivity and Lung Cancer

Different mutagens act on cells through different molecular mechanisms and so may activate different repair pathways. A person who is sensitive to one mutagen can be resistant to others (Hsu et al. 1993). Tobacco smoke contains a mixture of highly mutagenic compounds, such as polycyclic aromatic hydrocarbons; in particular, benzo[*a*]pyrene (B[*a*]P), a major constituent of tobacco smoke, has been reported to be one of the most potent carcinogenic compounds in vivo and in vitro (Hecht et al. 1993). The genotoxicity of B[*a*]P results from its in vivo metabolic activation by mammalian detoxification systems to highly reactive electrophilic diol epoxide metabolites, such as BPDE, that form covalent adducts upon interaction with DNA both in vitro and in vivo (Phillips 1983; Arce et al. 1987) and require excision repair (Tang et al. 1992; Van Houten et al. 1986). Moreover, strong and selective BPDE adduct formation occurred at *p53* hot spots (Denissenko et al. 1996). Therefore, measuring sensitivity to BPDE may shed some light on smoking-related cancer carcinogenesis. BPDE sensitivity might be a more relevant and more important assay for lung cancer.

We found (Table 1) that BPDE sensitivity was associated with a significantly elevated risk for lung cancer with an OR (95% CL) of 7.26 (3.00, 17.58), compared with an OR of 4.56 (1.91, 10.85) for bleomycin sensitivity for the same subjects (Wu et al. 1997). As with our data for bleomycin sensitivity, the ORs were even higher for lighter smokers and younger patients, supporting our hypothesis that mutagen sensitivity constitutes a susceptible phenotype. There was also a dose-response relationship between the quartiles of number of BPDE-induced breaks and lung cancer risk with ORs of 2.39, 3.12, and 15.03. We have also shown that age, sex, and smoking status do no independently modify the BPDE-sensitivity profile of cases and controls. This result is similar to a previous finding for bleomycin sensitivity (Wu et al. 1995). Interestingly, a significantly increased OR (95% CL) of 38.36 (9.83, 149.67) was noted for individuals who were sensitive to both

Table 1. Risk estimates of benzo[*a*]pyrene diol epoxide (*BPDE*) sensitivity in lung cancer patients and healthy controls (*OR* odds ratio; *CL* confidence limit)

BPDE sensitivity N (%)			Adjusted OR (CL)[a]	Adjusted OR (CL)[b]	Adjusted OR (CL)[c]
	Cases (51)	Controls (78)			
Breaks per cell					
≥0.58 (b/cell)	35 (68.63)	17 (21.79)	8.28 (3.65, 18.78)	8.86 (3.83, 20.47)	7.26 (3,00, 17.58)
<0.58 (b/cell)	16 (31.37)	61 (78.21)			
Cigarettes smoked/day					
<22 per day					
≥0.58 (b/cell)	22 (75.86)	8 (21.05)	12.74 (3.78, 42.96)	17.56 (4.47, 68.99)	14.47 (3.58, 58.59)
<0.58 (b/cell)	7 (24.14)	30 (78.95)			
22 + per day					
≥0.58 (b/cell)	13 (59.09)	9 (22.50)	5.30 (1.67, 16.78)	5.09 (1.53, 16.95)	4.91 (1.19, 20.27)
<0.58 (b/cell)	9 (40.91)	31 (77.50)			

[a] Adjusted by age and sex.
[b] Adjusted by age, sex, and pack-years.
[c] Adjusted by age, sex, pack-years, and bleomycin sensitivity.

BPDE and bleomycin. Thus, like bleomycin sensitivity, BPDE sensitivity can be used as a biological marker for identification of tobacco-susceptible individuals. BPDE sensitivity is a marker that reflects constitutional genetic instability. Bleomycin and BPDE sensitivity may represent two different major pathways or sensitivity pathways. These results provide strong support that individual sensitivity to BPDE may be associated with elevated risk of lung cancer. BPDE sensitivity may be a more relevant and more important susceptibility marker for lung cancer than bleomycin sensitivity.

BPDE specifically binds GC-rich and guanine-rich sequences of active genes and induces fragile sites (Popescu 1994). However, there is still little information on the molecular targets of the carcinogens in tobacco smoke. Mutagen-induced chromosomal breaks in a vital gene could induce expression of a quiescent oncogene or inactivate a tumor suppressor gene and thus lead to carcinogenesis. Therefore, searching for molecular targets of carcinogens in tobacco smoke will further our understanding of lung tumorigenesis.

Conclusion

Results from these studies indicate that variations in susceptibility to common mutagens contribute to lung cancer susceptibility. Results using bleomycin sensitivity as a measure of susceptibility to mutagens consistently show that this assay serves as a predictor of lung cancer risk. Bleomycin sensitivity is a general measure of DNA repair, which involves primarily DNA base excision repair mechanisms. Studies of BPDE-induced chromosomal breakage also demonstrate an association with lung cancer. This mutagen-based assay also serves as a measure of DNA repair activity, primarily through excision repair. Although these two mutagen-based assays measure different components of DNA repair, some components of the repair process may overlap. Study of the correlation between BPDE and bleomycin sensitivity to chromosomal damage shows a 46% correlation between these two biomarkers, indicating that 21% of the interindividual variation in BPDE sensitivity is explained by bleomycin sensitivity and vice versa. In addition to these global measures of DNA repair, studies to identify the specific components of DNA repair pathways that predispose to increased lung cancer risk are required. Other genetic factors have been suggested as contributors to lung cancer susceptibility. For instance, rather consistent increases in risk associated with glutathione-S-transferase null phenotype have been found (Strong and Amos 1996). Polymorphisms in cytochrome P450 enzymes, such as CYP2D6 and CYP1A1, have also shown an association with risk for lung cancer (Strong and Amos 1996). Large collaborative efforts are needed to accurately assess the independent effects of cytochrome P450s and other metabolizing enzymes.

In particular, the joint effects of both genetic and environmental agents have been predicted from segregation analyses to form the basis for common individual-specific sensitibity to lung cancer. An accurate assessment of how genetic and environmental agents interact to confer lung cancer sensitivity requires the development of large collaborative studies that share common protocols for the collection of critical epidemiological information such as smoking histories.

Acknowledgements. This work was supported by NIH grants CA 68437, CA 55769, CA 69089 and CA 95008. We would also like to thank Cynthia Thomas for secretarial and editorial assistance.

References

Aaltonen LA, Peltomaki P, Leach FS, Sistonen P, Pylkkanen L, Mecklin JP, Jarvinen H, Powel SM, Jen J, Hamilton SR, Petersen GM, Kinzler KW, Vogelstein B, de la Chapelle A (1993) Clues to the pathogenesis of familial colorectal cancer. Science 260:812–816

Arce GT, Allen JW, Doerr CL, Elmore E, Hatch GG, Moore MM, Shariet Y, Grunberger D, Nesnow S (1987) Relationships benzo(*a*)pyrene-DNA adducts levels and genotoxic effects in mammalian cells. Cancer Res 47:3388–3395

Bohr VA, Phillips DH, Hanawalt PC (1987) Heterogeneous DNA damage and repair in the mammalian genome. Cancer Res 47:6426–6436

Cloos J, Steen I, Joenje H, Ko JY, de Vries N, van der Sterre MLT, Nauta JJP, Snow GB, Braakhuis BJM (1993) Association between bleomycin genotoxicity and non-constitutional risk factors for head and neck cancer. Cancer Lett 74:161–165

Denissenko MF, Pao A, Tang M, Pfeifer GP (1996) Preferential formation of benzo[*a*]pyrene adducts at lung cancer mutational hotspots in p53. Science 274:430–432

Gauderman WJ, Morrison JL, Carpenter CL, Thomas DC (1997) Analysis of gene-smoking interaction in lung cancer. Genet Epidemiol 14:199–214

Glickman BN (1980) DNA repair and its relationship to the origins of human cancer. In: Cleton FJ, Simons JWIM (eds) Genetic origin of tumor cells. Nijhoff, The Hague, pp 25–51

Hecht SS, Carmella SG, Murphy SE, Foiles PG, Chung FL (1993) Carcinogen biomarkers related to smoking and upper aerodigestive tract cancer. J Cell Biochem Suppl 17 F:27–35

Hsu TC (1983) Genetic instability in the human population: a working hypothesis. Hereditas 98:1–9

Hsu TC, Johnston DA, Cherry LM, Ramkisson D, Schantz SP, Jessup JM, Winn RJ, Shirley L, Furlong C (1989) Sensitivity to geneotoxic effects of bleomycin in humans: possible relationship to environmental carcinogenesis. Int J Cancer 43:403–409

Hsu TC, Spitz MR, Schantz SP (1991) Mutagen sensitivity: a biologic marker of cancer susceptibility. Cancer Epidemiol Biomarkers Prev 1:83–89

Hsu TC, Feun I, Trizna Z, Savaraj N, Shirley L, Furlong CL, Schantz SP, Weber RS, Shen T, Hucuk O (1993) Differential sensitivity among three human subpopulations in response to 4-nitroquinoline-1-oxide and to bleomycin. Int J Oncol 3:827–830

Kawajiri K, Watanabe J, Eguchi H, Hayashi S (1995) Genetic polymorphisms of drug-metabolizing enzymes and lung cancer susceptibility. Pharmacogenetics 5:S70–73

Lee JJ, Trizna Z, Hsu TC, Spitz MR, Hong W (1996) A statistical analysis of the reliability and classification error in application of the mutagen sensitivity assay. Cancer Epidemiol Biomarkers Prev 5:191–197

McDuffie HH (1991) Clustering of cancer in families of patients with primary lung cancer. J Clin Epidemiol 44:69–76

Miki Y, Swensen J, Shattuck-Eidens D, Futreal PA, Harshman K, Tavtigian S, Liu Q, Cochran C, Bennett LM, Ding W, Bell R, Rosenthal J, Hussey C, Tran T, McClure M, Frye C, Hattier T, Phelps R, Haugen-Strano A, Katcher H, Yakumo K, Gholami Z, Shaffer D, Stone S, Bayer S, Wray C, Bogden R, Dayananth P, Ward J, Tonin P, Narod S, Bristo PK, Norris FH, Helvering I, Morrison P, Rosteck P, Lai M, Barrett JC, Lewis C, Neuhausen S, Cannon-Albright L, Goldgar D, Wieseman R, Kamb A, Skolnick MH (1994) A strong candidate for the breast and ovarian cancer susceptibility gene *BRACA 1*. Science 266:66–71

Nakachi K, Imai K, Hayashi S, Kawajiri K (1993) Polymorphisms of the *CYP 1 A 1* and gluthatione *S*-transferase genes associated with susceptibility to lung cancer in relation to cigarette dose in a Japanese population. Cancer Res 53:2994–2999

Nebert DW (1991) Role of genetics and drug metabolism in human cancer risk. Mutat Res 247:267–281

Ooi WL, Elston RC, Chen VW, Bailey-Wilson JE, Rothschild H (1986) Increased familial risk for lung cancer. J Natl Cancer Inst 76:217–222

Pandita TK, Hittelman WN (1995) Evidence of chromatin basis for increased mutagen sensitivity associated with multiple primary malignancies of the head and neck. Int J Cancer 61:738–743

Phillips DH (1983) Fifty years of benzo(*a*)pyrene (1983) Nature 303:468–472

Popescu NC (1994) Chromosome fragility and instability in human cancer. Crit Rev Oncog 5:121–140

Schantz SP, Spitz MR, Hsu TC (1990) Mutagen sensitivity in patients with head and neck cancers: a biologic marker for risk of multiple primary malignancies. J Natl Cancer Inst 82:1773–1775

Schwartz AG, Yang P, Swanson GM (1996) Familial risk of lung cancer among nonsmokers and their relatives. Am J Epidemiol 144:544–562

Sellers TA, Ooi WL, Elston RC, Chen VW, Bailey-Wilson JE, Rothschild H (1987) Increased familial risk for non-lung cancer among relatives of lung cancer patients. Am J Epidemiol 126:237–246

Sellers TA, Bailey-Wilson JE, Elston RC, Wilson AE, Rothschild H (1990) Evidence for Mendelian inheritance in the pathogenesis of lung cancer. J Natl Cancer Inst 82:1272–1279

Setlow RB (1978) Repair deficient human disorders and cancer. Nature 271:713–717

Spitz MR, Fueger JJ, Beddingfield NA, Annegers JF, Hsu TC, Newell GR, Schantz SP (1989) Chromosome sensitivity to bleomycin-induced mutagenesis, an independent risk factor for upper aerodigestive tract cancers. Cancer Res 49:4626–4628

Spitz MR, Fueger JJ, Halabi S, Schantz SP, Sample D, Hsu TC (1993) Mutagen sensitivity in upper aerodigestive tract cancer: a case-control analysis. Cancer Epidemiol Biomarkers Prev 2:329–333

Spitz MR, Hsu TC, Wu XF, Fueger JJ, Amos CI, Roth JA (1995) Mutagen sensitivity as a biologic marker of lung cancer risk in African-Americans. Cancer Epidemiol Biomarkers Prev 4:99–103

Strom SS, Wu XF, Sigurdson AJ, Hsu TC, Fueger JJ, Lopez J, Tee PG, Spitz MR (1995) Lung cancer, smoking patterns, and mutagen sensitivity in Mexican-Americans. J Natl Cancer Inst Monogr 18:29–33

Strong LC, Amos CI (1996) Inherited susceptibility. In: Schottenfeld D, Fraumeni JF Jr (eds) Cancer epidemiology and prevention. Oxford University Press, New York, pp 559–583

Tang MS, Pierce JR, Doisy RP, Nazimiec ME, Macleod MC (1992) Differences and similarities in the repair of two benzo[a]pyrene diol epoxide isomers induced DNA adducts by *uvrA, uvrB,* and *uvrC* gene products. Biochemistry 31:8429–8436

Tokuhata GK, Lillienfeld AM (1963) Familial aggregation of lung canncer in humans. J Natl Cancer Inst 30:289–312

Van Houten B, Masker WE, Carrier WL, Regan JD (1986) Quantitation of carcinogen-induced DNA damage and repair in human cells with the UVR ABC excision nuclease from *Escherichia coli.* Carcinogenesis 7:83–87

Wei Q, Spitz MR, Gu J, Cheng L, Xu X, Strom SS, Kripke ML, Hsu TC (1996) DNA repair capacity correlates with mutagen sensitivity in lymphoblastoid cell lines. Cancer Epidemiol Biomarkers Prev 5:199–204

Wu X, Delclos GL, Annegers JF, Bondy ML, Honn SE, Henry B, Hsu TC, Spitz MR (1995) A case-control study of wood dust exposure, mutagen sensitivity, and lung cancer risk. Cancer Epidemiol Biomarkers Prev 4:583–588

Wu XF, Shi H, Jiang H, Kemp B, Hong WK, Delclos GL, Spitz MR (1997) Associations between cytochrome P450E1 genotype, mutagen sensitivity, cigarette smoking and susceptibility to lung cancer. Carcinogenesis 18:967–973

Yang P, Schwartz AG, Mcallister AE, Aston CE, Swanson GM (1997) Genetic analysis of families with nonsmoking lung cancer probands. Genet Epidemiol 14:181–197

Yunis JJ, Soreng AL, Bowe AE (1987) Fragile sites are targets of diverse mutagens and carcinogens. Oncogene 1:59–69

Chemoprevention of Head and Neck and Lung (Pre)Cancer

N. de Vries[1], N. van Zandwijk[2] and U. Pastorino[3]

[1] Department of Otolaryngology/Head and Neck Surgery, Sint Lucas Andreas Hospital, location Lucas, Jan Tooropstraat 164, 1061 AE, Amsterdam, The Netherlands
[2] Netherlands Cancer Institute Amsterdam, The Netherlands
[3] Royal Brompton Hospital, London, England

Abstract

Oral cancer is often preceded by precancerous lesions, the most common of which is leukoplakia. Several treatment modalities are available: elimination of the possible cause, cold knife, laser, or cryosurgery, and topical application of bleomycin and 5-fluorouracil. In research, oral leukoplakia is used as a model to study the value of chemoprevention as a strategy to prevent cancer, because its effect is directly visible and material for analysis is easily obtainable from the mouth. In several studies and chemoprevention trials the efficacy of retinoids, retinol and/or beta-carotene on oral leukoplakia has been demonstrated. Second primary tumors occur in 10–30% of head and neck cancer patients and 10% of lung cancer patients. Chemoprevention offers an attractive approach to combat this threast to such patients, which is bound to cast a shadow over their lives. In the last 10–15 years several chemoprevention studies with vitamin A, retinoids or agents working through other mechanisms (antioxidants) have been launched. The largest chemoprevention study in curatively treated early-stage oral cancer, laryngeal cancer and lung cancer ($N = 2595$) is EUROSCAN, an EORTC study initiated in 1988. End-points are second tumors, local/regional recurrence and distant metastases, and long-term survival rates. Preminary results will be available in 1998.

Introduction

This paper focuses on work performed on chemoprevention of head and neck (pre)cancer and lung cancer. The emphasis will be on head and neck pathology. Head and neck cancer (oral cancer in particular, laryngeal cancer to a lesser extent) is preceded by precancerous lesions in a large proportion of cases.

Of the oral precancerous lesions, leukoplakia is by far the most common. Oral leukoplakia was defined by the World Health Organization Collaborating Centre for Oral Precancerous Lesions in 1978 as "a white patch or plaque

Recent Results in Cancer Research, Vol. 151
Senn/Costa/Jordan (Eds.): Chemoprevention of Cancer
© Springer-Verlag Berlin · Heidelberg 1999

that cannot be characterized clinically or pathologically as any other disease." In 1994 Axell et al., an international working group, rephrased the definition as „a predominantly white lesion of the oral mucosa that cannot be characterized as any other definable lesion", adding: "some oral leukoplakias will transform into cancer." A distinction is made between a provisional (clinical) and a definitive diagnosis. The definitive diagnosis or oral leukoplakia is a result of the identification and, if possible, elimination of suspected etiological factors, and in the case of persistent lesions – present for more than 2–4 weeks – pathological examination to rule out any other definalbe lesion and to determine the degree of epithelial dysplasias, if present. Erythroplakia, a red velvety plaque caused by epithelial thinning and dysplasia, and the admixed form erythroleukoplakia, are much less common. The prevalence of oral leukoplakia ranges from 1% to 10% in the adult population in the Western world. The age of the patients is usually above the fourth to fifth decade. In several studies a slight preference for occurrence in men is observed. There are not distinct racial differences. The use of tobacco in its various forms is considered to be the main etiologic factor. There are no data indicating an important role of nutrient intake with regard to oral (pre)cancer.

Two clinical types of oral leukoplakia are recognized, the homogeneous and the nonhomogeneous types. In general, biopsy is recommended in every case of oral leukoplakia. In homogeneous leukoplakia hyperkeratosis without epithelial dysplasia is the prevailing histological finding, while epithelial dysplasia, carcinoma in situ and even frank squamous cell carcinoma are more common histological findings in nonhomogeneous leukoplakia.

The prevalence of oral leukoplakia was studied by Hogewind and van der Waal (1988) in 1000 patients in The Netherlands. In a recent prevalence study of oral leukoplakia conducted by the same group (Schepman et al. 1996) using the new definition given above, prevalences of 0.6% and 0.2% were found for the provisional and the definitive diagnosis of oral leukoplakia, respectively. Malignant transformation of oral leukoplakia (Hogewind and van der Waal 1988), if it is untreated, takes place in 5–10% of all cases. In other series varying frequencies of 0.5–23% have been reported, depending on different inclusion criteria, geography and length of follow-up. The risk of such transformation is higher in leukoplakia (Lind 1987), and higher in erythroplakia than in leukoplakia. Furthermore, transformation to cancer occurs slightly more often in women than in men. The tongue and the floor of the mouth are the sites at risk, although malignant transformation can also occur in leukoplakias at other sites. Malignant transformation occurs almost exclusively in cases in which epithelial dysplasia has been observed in the biopsy. Spontaneous regression was hardly ever observed in this series, but has been reported in several others.

At present, several treatment modalities are available. In cases in which there is no clinical suspicion of cancer the primary treatment of leukoplakia is aimed at elimination of the possible cause. When no causative factors seem to be present or when no regression is obtained within 2–3 months after the elimination of such factor(s), further diagnotic work-up and treatment are indicated.

In the case of a solitary leukoplakia less than 2–3 cm in diameter an excisional biopsy can be performed. Performance of an incisional biopsy followed by cold knife surgery, laser surgery or cryosurgery is another common modality. Topical bleomycin and 5-fluorouracil have also been shown to be effective. Active treatment is always required in the presence of epithelial dysplasia, especially when the dysplasia is moderate or severe. The use of chemopreventive agents does not seem to be indicated in solitary, small leukoplakias.

In the case of multiple or extensive (larger than 2–3 cm) leukoplakias, in which one or more biopsies have not shown the presence of epithelial dysplasia, a wait-and-see policy can be followed. Of course, such a policy carries the potential risk of malignant transformation within a period of several months to several years. This is especially true for multiple or extensive leukoplakias, sometimes with ill-defined margins, in which the presence of moderate or severe epithelial dysplasia has been demonstrated and in which removal by cold knife surgery or laser evaporization is not possible. The potential value of chemoprevention of oral leukoplakia is particularly great in these patients with multiple and/or extensive lesions, irrespective of the presence of epithelial dysplasia. Since, in general, surgical excision allows recurrence in up to one third of cases, the place of adjuvant chemopreventive intervention (Chiesa et al. 1990, 1992, 1993) after treatment of oral leukoplakia is also being studied.

Patients with premalignant lesions in the head and neck not only have a higher risk that malignancy will occur at the site of the premalignant lesion; it has also been observed that the chance of a malignancy developing at other sites in the upper aerodigestive tract is also increased (de Vries 1990). From a research point of view, oral leukoplakia is regarded as the ideal model to study the value of chemoprevention as a strategy to prevent cancer in these tracts, because the effect of intervention is directly visible and material for analysis can easily be obtained from the site of the disease.

Chemoprevention of Oral Leukoplakia: Studies and Trials

Several studies and chemoprevention trials have demonstrated the efficacy of retinoids, retinol and/or beta carotene in reversing oral leukoplakia (Table 1). Although other interesting nonretinoid chemopreventive agents are being tested in chemoprevention trials by other study groups, they are not presently used in leukoplakia trials.

Table 1. Chemoprevention studies in oral leukoplakia (*%PR* partial response, *%CR* complete response, *%OR* % overall response, 13-*cis*-RA 13-*cis*-retinoic acid (isotretinoin), @@ randomisation to 20 mg fenretinide or no intervention after laser excision of the lesion)

Authors	Year	N	Drug	%CR	%PR	%OR
Silverman et al.	1963	16	Retinol, local	25	18	43
Raque et al.	1975	5	Tretinoin	20	80	100
Koch	1978	24	14-*cis*-RA	0	87	87
		24	Etretinatae	0	91	91
		27	Tretinoin	0	59	59
Koch	1981	24	Etretinate; oral, local	29	54	83
		21	Etretinate	24	47	71
Cordero et al.	1981	3	Etretinate	33	66	100
Shah et al.	1983	11	13-*cis*-RA, local	27	73	100
Hong et al.	1986	24	13-*cis*-RA	8	58	66
Stich et al.	1988	27	Beta carotene	15	?	15+?
		51	Beta carotene+Vit A	27	?	27+?
Stich et al.	1988	21	Vitamin A	57	?	57+?
Lippman et al.	1990	56	13-*cis*-RA/13-*cis*/RA/ beta carotene	13	49	62
Garewal et al.	1990	24	Beta carotene	8	63	71
Toma et al.	1990	15	Beta carotene	–	27	27
Toma et al.	1992	16	13-*cis*-RA 0.2 –> 1.0	7	29	36
Chiesa et al.	1992	115	Fenretinide (4-HPR) after laser surgery	@@		

Retinoids

Silverman et al. (1963) were the first to administer topical vitamin A in doses of 300 000–900 000 IU, to oral leukoplakia patients for 1–15 weeks, with responses in 43%. All patients had relapses after cessation of treatment. The lower dose (300 000 IU) was as effective as the dose of 900 000 IU. Koch, in 1978, randomized 72 patients into three groups: isotretinoin (13-*cis*-retinoic acid), tretinoin (beta-all-*trans* retinoic acid) and etretinate (an aromatic ethyl ester derivative). Objective (all partial) responses in the three groups occurred in 59–91%. This treatment was associated with considerable cutaneous and mucosal toxicity, and many relapses occurred after treatment was stopped. Later, several other nonrandomized studies yielded comparable responses with these same retinoids (Table 1).

Hong et al. (1986) performed the first double-blind phase III trial. Patients ($N=44$) were randomized to either placebo or isotretinoin, 1–2 mg/kg per day for 3 months. The response to isotretinoin was 67% (8% complete, 59% partial) in 24 patients versus a 10% (PR in 2 patients) response to placebo. No differences in responses between the doses of 1 and 2 mg/kg were found, but the mucocutaneous toxicity with the dose of 2 mg/kg was significant and occurred in 79% of patients. In Milan, Italy, 4-fenretinide (HPR) is being used after laser evaporization of oral leukoplakia to prevent local relapses and new localizations (Chiesa et al. 1990, 1992, 1993). The preliminary results do indeed point to chemopreventive activity. 4-HPR, which is also being used in an ongoing breast cancer chemoprevention trial at the same institute, is of particular interest, since it has no skin or mucosal toxicity. Finally, Lippman et al. (1993) conducted a study in which isotretinoin 1.5 mg/kg per day for 3 months was used for induction, after which patients were randomized to low-dose isotretinoin (0.5 mg/kg per day) or beta carotene at 30 mg per day. The response during induction therapy was 62%. Responses at the end of the maintenance phase showed isotretinoin to be more effective than beta carotene. Of particular interest was the observation that the toxicity of low-dose isotretinoin was no different from that of beta carotene.

Beta Carotene and Vitamin A

Stich's group (Stich et al. 1982, 1984, 1986, 1988; Stich and Rosin 1984) have conducted a number of studies in India in betel-nut chewers, a group with a high frequency of leukoplakia, using vitamin A alone or vitamin A and beta carotene together. In 1988 Stich et al. randomized 130 patients to placebo, beta carotene 180 mg/week, and beta carotene 180 mg/week with vitamin A 100 000 IU/week. At 6 months, complete responses rates were 3%, 15% and 28%, respectively. New lesions were better suppressed in the combined treatment group than in the two other groups: 8% versus 15% and 21% (placebo). In a second randomized trial, patients received placebo or vitamin A, 200 000 IU/week for 6 months. A 57% complete remission (CR) rate and complete suppression of new lesions occurred in the treatment group, as opposed to a 3% CR rate and 21% with new lesions in the placebo arm. Although it must be realized that this study population is different from that the lesions have been caused by tobacco and betel-nut chewing, it is noteworthy that these responses are the best of all reported in the various studies.

Garewal et al. in 1990 treated 24 patients with beta carotene, 30 mg/day for 3 months. Seventeen (71%) patients has responses, 2 of them complete responses. Toma et al. (1990), however, using beta carotene 90 mg/day for 6 months found responses in only 27% of 24 patients.

Biomarkers as Intermediate Endpoints as Applicable to Leukoplakia

Leukoplakia is not only regarded as an ideal model in which to test chemoprevention; it is used in particular for testing biomarkers as intermediate endpoints. Chemoprevention has a serious problem with regard to the feasibility of the conduct of clinical trials. Investigators are still forced to rely on cancer incidence as the study endpoint. The corollary of this is that chemoprevention trials require many more patients and longer follow-up periods and also involve much higher costs than standard phase III chemotherapy trials (Lippman et al. 1990). There is therefore a need for a process to establish optimal drugs, doses and duration of administration to solve the problems of the high number of patients and the enormous amount of time and money involved, and is felt that intermediate endpoints would make prevention trials (more) feasible. This field of research involves biomarkers as intermediate endpoints of carcinogenesis. It is hoped that their use will lead to the development of cost-effective trials. Biomarkers include clinical markers, histological markers and cytological markers. Chemoprevention trials require markers that reveal early carcinogenic changes and yield information about the risk on malignant transformation. An ideal biomarker should meet the following requirements: (1) predict response to chemoprevention, (2) allow monitoring of chemopreventive treatment, (3) be of value in selection of new chemopreventive agents (4) indicate level of risk of malignant transformation. With all this in view, Copper et al. (1993) investigated the value of a panel of monoclonal antibodies to identify biomarkers in the oral mucosa that are associated with cancer risk. As a model, the expression of antigens was assessed in cytological preparations obtained from macroscopically normal oral mucosa of patients with a tongue carcinoma and of controls. The panel included antibodies against cytokeratin 8, 10, 13 and 19. In oral mucosa of cancer patients the expression of cytokeratin 19 was over 3 times that in controls, which makes it an interesting candidate as an intermediate endpoint.

Once good biomarkers were found, more chemoprevention trials could then be carried out in less time and with fewer patients. With respect to chemoprevention trials in leukoplakia, an efficient use of patients eligible for such intervention is in particular warranted since these patients are relatively rare, as reflected (Table 1) by the small series of patients enrolled in chemoprevention trials and studies in oral leukoplakia.

In conclusion, only a minority of oral leukoplakia patients are candidates for therapeutic treatment with chemopreventive agents. Treatment begins with the elimination of etiologic factors. In solitary leukoplakias less than 2–3 cm in diameter, surgery in its various forms, topical bleomycin and 5-fluorouracil can be applied. A wait-and-see policy is also followed. The value of chemoprevention is greatest in patients with multiple and/or extensive lesions. Leukoplakia recurs after surgical excision in one third of cases. Therefore, adjunctive chemopreventive intervention might also have a role. Although it is attractive from a research point of view to treat leukoplakia with chemopreventive agents, this is not indicated in all patients. At present there is little place for routine use of chemopreventive agents. At present, patients should preferably be entered in (multicenter) clinical trials, since the ideal chemopreventive agent (or combination) and the best dosage and treatment schedule have still to be established. Such studies, can also be the background to research into biomarkers as intermediate endpoints. Responses for the three retinoids studied: isotretinoin (13-*cis*-retinoic acid), tretinoin and etretinate, are comparable. Most experience has been recorded with 13-*cis*-retinoic acid, which produces remissions in 65–80% of cases. Unfortunately,

13-*cis*-retinoic acid at high doses has severe toxicity. Vitamin A 200 000 IU/ week produced the highest complete response (57%) reported. In this connection, it is of interest that the toxicity of vitamin A, even in doses of 300 000/day for 2 years, as in the EUROSCAN trial (see below), is in general mild and well tolerated (de Vries et al. 1991). It is not clear, however, whether the responses to vitamin A found in betel-nut chewers in India can be extrapolated to the idiopathic or tobacco-induced leukoplakia cases seen in the Western world. In several studies mentioned the patients were not optimally defined, which might possibly have led to a bias with regard to treatment responses. With all drugs and in all studies, many lesions recurred when treatment was discontinued.

Chemoprevention of Laryngeal (Pre)Cancer

Laryngeal squamous cell hyperplasia (leukoplakia) is a precursor of laryngeal cancer. A unknown proportion of laryngeal cancers develop out of these hyperplasias. The laryngeal hyperplasias can be divided into three groups according to Kleinsasser (1988): simple hyperplasia (class I), moderate dysplasia (class II) and carcinoma in situ (class III). The higher the class, the higher the potential for malignant transformation. There also appears to be a tendency to develop more second tumors elsewhere in the upper aerodigestive system, with a preference for the lung, with higher classes, as in invasive laryngeal cancer. In two series the incidence of second tumors in laryngeal squamous cell hyperplasia was 10–21.9% (de Vries et al. 1986; Lundgren and Olofsson 1987). The chance of developing additional tumors is therefore almost as high as in invasive laryngeal cancer. Recently, in the first study on chemoprevention of laryngeal squamous cell hyperplasia with retinol palmitate in an induction phase dose of 300 000 IU, or more in the case of resistant lesions, and a later maintenance phase of 150 000 IU, 15 of 20 cases achieved complete response (Issing et al. 1997). In the other 5 patients partial remission was seen. Videostroboscopy, allows accurate monitoring of response to chemoprevention in laryngeal hyperplasia. The only drawback of this model, compared with oral leukoplakia, is the difficulty of taking repeated biopsies at the site of the lesion.

Chemoprevention of Head and Neck Cancer

Second primary tumors occur in 10–30% of head and neck cancer and 10% of lung cancer patients. The majority of these second cancers occur again in the head and neck or in the lungs and the esophagus, and they often have a poor prognosis. Two approaches have been investigated to combat the problem of second tumors in head and neck cancer patients: early detection and (chemo-)prevention. Regarding early detection, it has become common prac-

Table 2. Chemoprevention trials in head and neck cancer

Institute	Year	Stages	Site[a]	Drug/Dose	N	RES
M.D. Anderson	1984–1990	All	All	13-*cis*-RA 50–100 mg/m^2	103	+
Gettec	1985–1991	Early	Mouth, oropharynx	Etretinate 50–>25 mg	323	–
EUROSCAN	1988–1996	Early	Mouth, larynx, lung	RP 300 000 IU, NAC 600 mg	2532	?
CONNECTICUT	1990–>	Early	All	Beta carotene, 50 mg	600	?
M.D. Anderson	1991–>	Early	All	13-*cis*-RA 30 mg/m^2	1000	?
EUROSCAN II	1998 (?)	Early	All	To be announced	?	?

[a] All sites: mouth, oro- and hypopharynx, and larynx.

tice at many centers to perform panendoscopy during the initial work-up of head and neck cancer patients. However, most second tumors occur metachronously, and it has been shown that regular endoscopic investigation – e.g. half-year panendoscopy or bronchoscopy – is not feasible. As a result, many second tumors are still not detected until they are beyond a curable stage during follow-up.

Chemoprevention offers a more attractive approach to combating this "overshadowing threat" to early-stage head and neck cancer patients. In the last 10–10 years, chemoprevention studies have been launched at several places throughout the world, with varying degrees of success. Many animal, in vitro and epidemiological studies have shown a protective effect of vitamin A and the retinoids. Several clinical chemoprevention trials with vitamin A, retinoids or agents working by way of other mechanisms (antioxidants) are also currently in progress (Table 2). Curatively treated and early-stage head and neck cancer and lung cancer patients are an ideal population to test the value of chemopreventive medication, because of the extremely high risk of developing second tumors. Chemoprevention may gradually be developing from its status as an interesting experimental modality to a realistic preventive measure as adjuvant treatment after head and neck cancer has once been cured.

Hong et al. (1990) published the results of their study in which 12-*cis*-retinoic acid (isotretinoin), 50–100 mg/m^2 body surface area for 12 months was used. In this study, in which 103 patients were entered, only 2 (4%) second tumors occurred in the isotretinoin group, as against to 12 (24%) in the placebo group. These data showed for the first time that chemoprevention of second tumors in head and neck cancer patients is possible. Unfortunately, however, the study has several drawbacks: the toxicity of 13-*cis*-retinoic acid in the dose used was considerable and defies further treatment in this dose. The number of patients in the study was limited and the number of second tumors in the untreated group (24%) after 32 months is exceptionally high, indeed higher than in almost any other retro- or prospective study reported in the literature. The possibility that the enormous difference between the two groups is due to chance cannot be disregarded. All stages of head and neck cancer patients were eligible, and not early-stage patients only. In a later follow-up (median 54.5 months) report Benner et al. (1994) showed that the number of second tumors increased in both groups, to 14% vs 32%, indicating that a delay in occurrence had been reached rather than permanent prevention. In an ongoing study by the same group a lower dose of 13-*cis*-retinoic acid is being investigated in a larger number of early-stage patients only.

In the Frence Gettec study reported by Bolla et al. (1994), 323 patients with early stage (T 1–2, N0-1) oral cavity and oropharynx tumors were randomized to placebo or etretinate at a dose of 50 mg/day in the 1st month and 25 mg/day in the subsequent 23 months. There were no significant differences in loco-regional and distant relapse or second primary tumors. The 5-year survival was 64% in the etretinate group and 75% in the placebo group.

By far the largest chemoprevention study in head and neck cancer patients is EUROSCAN. EUROSCAN is a European chemoprevention study in curatively treated early stage oral cancer, laryngeal cancer and lung cancer patients, which was initiated in 1988 under the aegis of the European Organization of Research and Treatment of Cancer (EORTC). The patients receive retinyl palmitate, 300 000 IU daily for 1 year and half this dose during a 2nd year, or *N*-acetylcysteine (NAC), 600 mg for 2 years, or both drugs or neither, in a 2×2 factorial design. NAC has shown positive chemopreventive activity in all animal models tested (de Flora et al. 1986; Wilpart et al. 1986; Cesarone et al. 1987; Rothstein and Slaga 1988; Boone et al. 1992).

Between 1988 and 1994, 2595 patients were randomized (1076 larynx, 490 oral and 1029 lung cancer patients). Endpoints are second tumors, local/regional recurrence and distant metastases, and long-time survival rates. A first analysis of the treatment effects is expected in late 1998 or early 1999.

Most (93%) of the subjects in the EUROSCAN population were regular smokers. The oral cancer group contained more nonsmokers than the groups with cancer in other sites. The median age at the start of regular smoking was 17 years. Half the patients in the study had an exposure of at least 43 pack-years. Both sex and age were strongly related to aspects of smoking behavior, i.e. filter cigarettes were the favorite type of cigarette among females and the youngest members of the population. The data suggest that filter cigarettes were related to different sites of disease than non filter cigarettes: nonfilter cigarettes were more frequently recorded in the history of patients with laryngeal cancer than in that of patients with lung cancer. Sixteen percent of the patients continued to smoke after the diagnosis of first malignancy. Although the frequency and intensity of side effects of preventive medication do not seem to be related to the continuation of smoking, a negative effect of continuation of smoking on survival is suggested. An intermediate analysis of side effects and toxicity in the EUROSCAN patients has shown that both the single-drug treatment and the combination treatment are mostly well tolerated and that the toxicity is mild, comparing favorably with that of the intervention used by Hong et al. (1990). Skin dryness and desquamation were the most frequent symptoms, affecting 60% of the patients treated. Other symptoms, such as dyspepsia, headache, nosebleeds and mild hair loss, occurred in under 10% of patients and cleared up without treatment.

Jyothirmayi et al. (1996), in India, evaluated the effectiveness of vitamin A in preventing local relapses and second tumors in a randomized trial involving 106 patients. Patients were randomized to retinyl palmitate (200 000 IU per week for 1 year) or placebo. One fifth (11/56) of the patients in the treated group and one tenth (5/50) in the placebo group had loco-regional recurrence. No second primaries were observed in the vitamin A group, though 2 patients in the placebo group had second tumors. The higher frequency of recurrences in the vitamin A group concerned the authors, although they correctly stated that the small size of the trial could account for the finding. The study was mainly conducted as a pilot study to evaluate patient compliance, acceptability of supplements, and the feasibility of adequate follow-up.

Chemoprevention of Lung Cancer

Pastorino et al. (1988, 1991, 1993) were the first to report on chemoprevention of curatively resected stage I lung cancer. Retinyl palmitate (300 000 IU daily for at least 12 months) administration was used as adjuvant treatment. After a median follow-up of 28 months, 283 patients could be evaluated: 138 allocated to treatment with retinyl palmitate and 145 to standard treatment. In 113 (37%) patients new tumor growth was observed: 47 (31%) in the intervention arm and 66 (42%) in the control arm ($P = 0.051$). In total, 35 second primary tumors in 32 patients occurred: 14 (9%) in the intervention arm and 21 (13%) in the controls.

Recently, disappointing results of large-scale primary intervention trials with beta carotene have been published (Alpha-Tocopherol, Beta Carotene Cancer Prevention Study Group 1994). In a Finnish primary prevention study (1994), 29 133 heavy smokers were randomized into four groups receiving one, both, or neither of 50 mg alpha tocopherol (vitamin E) and 20 mg beta carotene per day. In the beta carotene group 18% more lung cancer (statistically significant) and 8% more mortality was found. In the Physicians Health Study (Alpha Tocopherol, Beta Carotene Cancer Prevention Study Group 1994), 22 071 male American doctors participated: 11 036 took beta carotene 50 mg and 11 035, placebo. In the beta carotene group 1273 malignancies occurred, as against 1293 in the placebo group. In the beta carotene group 82 lung cancers were observed, as against 88 lung cancers in the placebo group (not significant). In the CARET study (Hennekens et al. 1996) 18 314 women and men at high risk – smokers and persons exposed to asbestos – participated. A combination of beta carotene (30 mg) and retinol (25 000 IU/day was used). The treated group had 28% more lung cancers and a 17% higher mortality than the placebo group (not significant).

References

Alpha-Tocopherol, Beta Carotene Cancer Prevention Study Group (1994) The effect of vitamin E and beta carotene on the incidence of lung cancer and other cancers in male smokers. N Engl J Med 330:1029–1035

Axell T, Pindborg JJ, Smith CJ, van der Waal I and an International Collaborative Group on Oral White Lesions (1996) Oral white lesions with special reference to precancerous and tobacco-related lesions: conclusion of a international symposium held in Uppsala, Sweden. J Oral Pathol Med 25:49–54

Benner SE, Pajak TF, Lippman SM, Earley C, Hong WK (1994) Prevention of second primary tumors with isotretinoin in patients with squamous cell carcinoma of the head and neck: long term follow-up. J Natl Cancer Inst 86:140–141

Bolla M, Lefus R, Ton Van J et al (1994) Prevention of second primary tumors with etretinate in squamous cell carcinoma of oral cavity and oropharynx. Results of a multicentric double-blind randomized study. Cancer Res 54:854–856

Boone CW, Steele VE, Kelloff GJ (1992) Screening for chemopreventive (anticarcinogenic) compounds in rodents. Mutat Res 267:251–255

Cesarone CF, Scarabelli L, Orenesu M, Bagnasco M, De Flora S (1987) Effects of aminothiols in 2-acetylaminofluorone-treated rats. I. Damage and repair of liver DNA, hyperplastic foci, and Zymbal gland tumors. In Vivo 1:85–91

Chiesa F, Tradati N, Sala L et al (1990) Follow-up of oral leukoplakia after carbon dioide laser surgery. Arch Otolaryngol Head Neck Surg 116:177–181

Chiesa F, Tradati N, Marazzi M et al (1992) Prevention of local relapses and new localizations of oral leukoplakias with the synthetic retinoid fenretinide (4-HPR). Preliminary results. Oral Oncol Eur J Cancer 24 B:97–102

Chiesa F, Tradati N, Rossi N et al (1993) Fenretinide (4-HPR) in chemoprevention of oral leukoplakia. J Cell Biochem Suppl 17 F:255–261

Copper MP, Braakhuis BJM, de Vries N, van Dongen GAMS, Nauta JP, Snow GB (1993) A panel of biomarkers of carcinogenesis of the upper aerodigestive tract as potential intermediate end points in chemoprevention trials. Cancer 71:825–830

Cordero AA, Allevato MAJ, Barclay CA et al (1981) Retinoids: advances in basis research and therapy. Springer, Berlin Heidelberg New York, p 273

De Flora s, Astengo M, Serra D, Benicelli C (1986) Prevention of induced lung tumors in mice by dietary N-acetylcysteine. Cancer Lett 32:235–241

De Vries N (1990) The magnitude of the problem. In: de Vries N, Gluckman JL (eds) Multiple primary tumors in the head and neck. Thieme, Stuttgart, pp 1–25

De Vries N, Oldekalter P, Snow GB (1986) Multiple primary tumors in patients with laryngeal squamous cell hyperplasia. Arch Otorhinolaryngol 243:143–145

De Vries N, van Zandwijk N, Pastorino U (1991) The EUROSCAN Trial (Guest Editorial). Br J Cancer 64:985–989

Garewal Hs, Meyskens FL, Killen D, Reeves D, Kiersch TA, Elletson H, Strosberg A, King D, Streinbronn K (1990) Response of oral leukoplakia to beta-carotene. J Clin Oncol 8:1715–1720

Hennekens CH, Buring JE, Manson JE, Stampher M, Rosner B, Cook NR et al (1996) Lack of effect of long term supplementation with beta carotene on the incidence of malignant neoplasms and cardiovascular disease. N Engl J Med 334:1145–1149

Hogewind WFC, van der Waal I (1988) Prevalence study of oral leukoplakia in a selected population of 1000 patients from the Netherlands. Community Dent Epidemiol 16:302–305

Hong WK, Endicott J, Itri L (1986) 13-cis retinoic acid in the treatment of oral leukoplakia. N Engl J Med 315:1501–1505

Hong WK, Lippman SM, Itri LM, Karp DD, Lee JS, Byers RM, Schantz SP, Kramer AM, Lotan R, Peters LJ, Dimery IW, Brown BW, Goepfert H (1990) Prevention of second tumors with isotretinoin in squamous-cell carcinoma of the head and neck. N Engl J Med 323:795–801

Issing WJ, Struck R, Naumann A (1997) Positive impact of retinyl palmitate in leukoplakia of the larynx. Eur Arch Otorhinolaryngol 254:105–109

Jyothirmayi R, Ramadas K, Varghese C, Jacob R, Nair MK, Sankaranarayanan R (1996) Efficacy of vitamin A in the prevention of loco-regional recurrence and second primaries in head and neck cancer. Oral Oncol Eur J Cancer 6:373–376

Kleinsasser O (1988) Precancerous lesions. In: Kleinsasser O (ed) Tumors of the larynx and hypopharynx. Thieme, Stuttgart, pp 61–69

Koch HF (1978) Biochemical treatment of precancerous oral lesions: the effectiveness of various analogues of retinoic acid. J Maxillofac Surg 6:59–63

Koch HF (1981) Advances in basic research and therapy. Springer, Berlin Heidelberg New York, pp 307–312

Lind PO (1987) Malignant transformation in oral leukoplakia. Scand J Dent Res 95:449–455

Lippman SM, Lee JS, Lotan R, Hittelman W, Wargovich MJ, Hong WK (1990) Biomarkers as intermediate endpoints in chemoprevention trials. J Natl Cancer Inst 82:555–560

Lippman SM, Batsakis, Toth BB et al (1993) Comparison of low-dose isotretinoin with beta-carotene to prevent oral carcinogenesis. N Engl J Med 328:15–20

Lundgren J, Olofsson J (1987) Malignant tumours in patients with non-invasive squamous cell lesions of the vocal cords. Clin Otolaryngol 12:39–43

Omenn GS, Goodman GE, Thornquist MD, Balmes J, Cullen Mr, Glass A et al (1996) Effects of a combination of beta carotene and vitamin A on lung cancer and cardiovascular disease in asbestos-exposed workers and in smokers. N Engl J Med 334:1150–1155

Pastorino U, Soresi E, Clerici M, Chiesa G, Belloni PA, Ongari M, Valente M, Ravasi G (1988) Lung cancer chemoprevention with Retinol Palmitate. Acta Oncol 27:1–10

Pastorino U, Chiesa G, Infante M, Soresi E, Clerici M, Valente M, Belloni PA, Ravasi G (1991) Safety of high dose vitamin A. Oncology 48:131–137

Pastorino U, Infante M, Maioli M, Chiesa G, Buyse M, Firket P, Rosmentz N, Clerici M, Soresi E, Valente M, Belloni PA, Ravasi G (1993) Adjuvant treatment of stage I lung cancer with high dose vitamin A. J Clin Oncol 11:1216–1222

Raque CJ, Biondo RV, Keeran MG et al (1975) Snuff dippers' keratosis (snuff-induced leukoplakia). South Med 68:565–568

Rothstein JB, Slaga TJ (1988) Effect of exogenous glutathione on tumour progression in the murine skin multistage carcinogenesis model. Carcinogenesis 9:1547–1551

Schepman KP, van der Meij EH, Smeele LF, van der Waal I (1996) Prevalence study or oral white lesions with special reference to a new definition of oral leukoplakia. Oral Oncol Eur J Cancer 32 B:416–419

Shah JP, Strong EW, DeCosse JJ (1983) Effect of retinoids on oral leukoplakia. Am J Surg 146:466–470

Silverman S, Renstrup G, Pindborg JJ (1963) Studies in oral leukoplakias. Acta Odontol Scand 21:271–292

Stich HF, Rosin MP (1984) Micronuclei in exfoliated human cells as a tool for studies in cancer risk and cancer intervention. Cancer Lett 22:241–253

Stich HF, Stich W, Parida BB (1982) Elevated frequency of micronucleated cells in the buccal mucosa of individuals at high risk for oral cancer: betel quid chewers. Cancer Lett 17:125–134

Stich HF, Stich W, Rosin MP, Vallejera MO (1984) Use of the micronucleus test to monitor the effect of vitamin A, beta-carotene and canthaxanthin on the buccal mucosa of betel nut/tobacco chewers. Int J Cancer 34:745–750

Stich HF, Hornby AP, Dunn BP (1986) A pilot beta-carotene intervention trial in patients using smokeless tobacco. Int J Cancer 36:321–327

Stich HF, Hornby Ad, Mathew B (1988) Response of oral leukoplakias to the administration of vitamin A. Cancer Lett 40:93–101
Toma S, Albanese M, DeLorenzi G et al (1990) Beta-carotene in the treatment of oral leukoplakia. Proc Am Soc Clin Oncol 9:179
Toma S, Mangiante PE, Margariano G, Nicolo G, Palumbo R (1992) Progressive 13-*cis*-retinoic acid dosage in the treatment of oral leukoplakia. Oral Oncol J Cancer 24 B121–123
Wilpart M, Speder A, Roberfroid M (1986) Anti-initiation activity of N-acetyl-cysteine in experimental colonic carcinogenesis. Cancer Lett 31:319–324
World Health Organization Collaborating Centre for Oral Precancerous Lesions (1978) Definition of leukoplakia and related lesions: an aid to studies on oral precancer. Oral Surg 46:518–539

II. Targets and Markers
for Cancer Prevention

Rationale and Mechanisms of Cancer Chemoprevention

S. De Flora, C. Bennicelli, and M. Bagnasco

Institute of Hygiene and Preventive Medicine, University of Genoa,
Via A. Pastore 1, I-16132 Genoa, Italy

Abstract

Chronic degenerative diseases, including cancer, have a multifactorial origin. An intricate network connects each disease with multiple risk factors and also with multiple protective factors. From the point of view of preventive medicine, this implies that removal of a single risk factor will have a beneficial impact on the epidemiology of several diseases. However, in contrast to the situation in infectious diseases, it will never be possible to eradicate any chronic degenerative disease in this way, because each of them is associated with other risk factors at the same time. Similarly, a single protective factor can decrease the risk of contracting different diseases, and the risk of developing a single disease can be attenuated by different protective factors, often in a coordinated fashion. It is thus evident that cancer can be prevented not only by avoiding exposure to recognized risk factors, but also, as a complementary approach referred to as chemoprevention, by favouring the intake of protective factors and by fortifying the physiological defences of the host organism. Chemoprevention can be applied in a primary prevention setting when it is addressed to healthy individuals with the goal of inhibiting occurrence of the disease. Conversely, it is applied in a secondary prevention setting when it is addressed to individuals affected by premalignant tumours, with the goal of reversing the carcinogenesis process. A rational use of chemopreventive agents is based not only on the assessment of their efficacy and safety but also on understanding of their mechanisms of action. A detailed classification is proposed, which covers a variety of mechanisms interfering with different phases of mutagenesis and carcinogenesis. However, this sequence of events does not fit in with a rigid scheme, and several mechanisms, such as inhibition of genotoxic effects, antioxidant activity and scavenging of free radicals, inhibition of cell proliferation, and signal transduction modulation are reiterated several times throughout evolution of these processes. Some of these mechanisms are also involved in advanced stages of tumour progression towards malignancy, invasion and metastasis, and can therefore conveniently be applied for the tertiary prevention of cancer. Most inhibitors work through multiple mechanisms, examples of which are given for 18 chemopreventive agents.

Recent Results in Cancer Research, Vol. 151
Senn/Costa/Jordan (Eds.): Chemoprevention of Cancer
© Springer-Verlag Berlin · Heidelberg 1999

Risk Factors and Protective Factors in Cancer Epidemiology

That there is a relationship between environment and human health has been known since ancient times. In fact, the man-environment binomial was described 2500 years ago by the Greek physician Hippocrates, the Father of Medicine, and thereafter identified as "Hippocrates' dyad". Following the discovery and characterization of pathogenic organisms from the late nineteenth century onward this dyad became a triad as the etiological agents that are the necessary yet not sufficient causes of infectious diseases were incorporated. Therefore, removal of an etiological agent will lead to eradication of the corresponding infectious condition, as has already occurred for several diseases on a regional scale and for smallpox on a worldwide scale.

Unfortunately, the situation is quite different for cancer and other chronic degenerative diseases. Rather than rigid associations between etiological agents and diseases, there is an intricate network connecting different risk factors and different chronic degenerative diseases. Owing to this multifactorial origin, avoidance of an individual risk factor may have a beneficial impact on the epidemiology of different diseases falling in this category, but will never succeed in their complete eradication, since each of them is associated with other risk factors at the same time.

Luckily, besides the epidemiology of risk factors there is also an epidemiology of protective factors, which again are connected in a multifactorial fashion with chronic degenerative diseases, and in turn each disease can be attenuated by different protective factors, which often work in combination. This is typical for complex mixtures such as foodstuffs, and is exploited in so-called combined chemoprevention (see below).

It is evident that the occurrence of cancer or other chronic degenerative diseases is just the visible tip of an iceberg, even though these are by far the most common causes of death in the population. The disease is the outcome of the balance of exposures to risk factors and protective factors, and of their impact and interplay with the physiological mechanisms of the host organism. Accordingly, prevention can be pursued either by minimizing exposures to risk factors or by favouring exposures to protective factors and fortifying the host defence mechanisms. The latter approach is referred to as chemoprevention.

The Three Levels of Prevention

In general, prevention can be applied at three levels, which correspond to consecutive steps along the natural history of a disease (Last 1986). In particular, *primary prevention* is prevention of the occurrence of a disease and is therefore directed at apparently healthy individuals, irrespective of the fact that they may be at high risk either because they have an enhanced individual susceptibility or because they are exposed to recognized risk factors.

Secondary prevention consists in early diagnosis, preferably at a preclinical stage, and it is therefore directed at individuals in whom the disease has already started its pathogenetic course but it is still in the latency period or at most in an early clinical phase. Clearly, early detection is followed by timely intervention aimed at reversing, halting, or at least retarding the progress of a condition. *Tertiary prevention* is aimed at preventing recurrences, further progression and complications and is therefore aimed at individuals who have been previously cured of a disease. Together with rehabilitation, this kind of intervention falls within the scope of patient management, and it is particularly relevant in the case of chronic degenerative diseases such as cancer, which often pose the problem of incomplete recovery and a trend to recurrences and complications.

Approaches to Cancer Prevention

Figure 1 shows the time-course of possible intervention strategies against cancer, as related to the different steps of the carcinogenesis process and to the growth patterns of the neoplastic mass. Starting from a single transformed cell, 30 cell doublings are needed to form a mass composed of 1 billion cells, weighing approximately 1 g. Depending on several factors, such as localization and accessibility of the tumour, education of the patient, and diagnostic possibilities, this may be the time for secondary prevention. Otherwise, with even a very few cell division the neoplastic mass will enlarge further with a tremendous growth acceleration. This explains the problems encountered in the treatment of cancer, especially those cancers in which an early diagnosis is hardly achievable and treatment is expected to be applied at a later stage, after invasion and metastasis of malignant cells. Tertiary prevention of cancer consists in the prevention of local recurrences and metastatic spread of metastases.

As previously discussed, primary prevention can be pursued by way of two complementary approaches: avoidance of exposure to recognized carcinogens and protection of the host organism. The former approach involves risk assessment followed by risk management. In particular, health education measures are aimed at reducing exposures to lifestyle risk factors, whereas suitable regulations are implemented to reduce exposures to environmental (in a strict sense) risk factors.

Objectives of Cancer Chemoprevention

Chemoprevention was defined by Sporn and Newton (1979) as the administration of agents to prevent induction, to inhibit, or to delay progression of cancers, and by Kelloff et al. (1994) as the inhibition or reversal of carcinogenesis at a premalignant stage. Therefore, as illustrated in Fig. 1, chemopre-

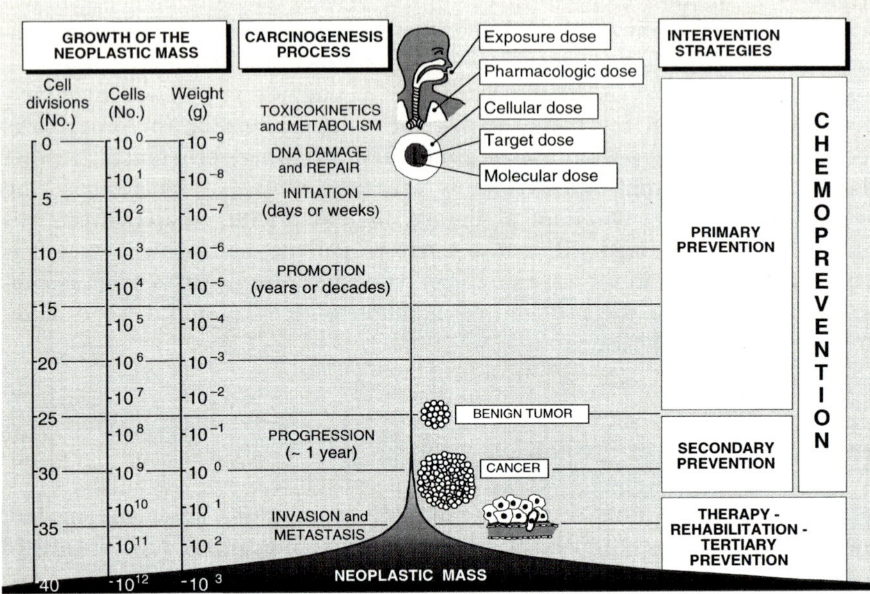

Fig. 1. Intervention strategies against cancer, as related to the carcinogenesis process and growth patterns of the neoplastic mass

vention is a part of primary prevention and complementary to the avoidance of exposure to recognized carcinogens, when it is addressed to healthy individuals with the goal of inhibiting carcinogenesis. Conversely, the reversal of carcinogenesis falls within secondary prevention, since it follows the early detection of premalignant lesions. Chemoprevention of second primaries, which is a frequent objective in clinical trials, can also be included under secondary prevention, since possible second primaries are expected to be latent when an intervention is carried out.

This distinction, which is frequently overlooked, is not merely academic. In fact, chemopreventive agents that are effective in a primary prevention setting are not necessarily effective in a secondary prevention setting, and vice versa. It should be noted that chemoprevention studies in animal models are usually designed to mimic the primary prevention of cancer, while most chemoprevention clinical trials evaluate the regression of premalignant lesions or prevention of second primaries, and accordingly fall within secondary prevention. Indeed, both prevention of cancer in healthy individuals and regression of lesions in individuals affected by premalignant forms are extremely important, yet different, objectives.

Mechanisms of Inhibitors of Mutagenesis and Carcinogenesis

For a rational implementation of chemoprevention it is essential not only to establish efficacy and safety or putative agents in vitro, in animal models and in clinical trials (Bertram et al. 1987; De Flora et al. 1992), but also to evaluate the mechanisms by which chemopreventive agents exert their protective effects. Once the mode of action of inhibitors is understood useful information becomes available for supporting or predicting efficacy, for delineating the field of application and targets of chemopreventive agents, and for designing suitable combinations of agents. Several examples are available of combinations of agents working through complementary mechanism (Kelloff and Boone 1994).

Most classifications of inhibitors take into account the multistep nature of the carcinogenesis process. Interestingly, it has been postulated that the diphasic initiation-promotion process leading to the formation of a benign neoplastic mass occurs in the pathogenesis not only of cancer but also of other chronic degenerative diseases (Trosko and Chang 1980; De Flora et al. 1996b). According to Wattenberg (1981), chemopreventive agents can be distinguished into blocking agents, which prevent carcinogens from reaching or reacting with critical target sites, and suppressing agents, which prevent the evolution of the neoplastic process. These agents are inhibitors of initiation and of promotion/progression, respectively (Morse and Stoner 1993). Inhibitors of mutagenesis were categorized by Kada et al. (1982) into desmutagens and bioantimutagens, which inactivate mutagens before they can attack DNA and interfere with fixation of DNA damage, respectively. The ICPEMC Expert Group of Antimutagens and Desmutagens proposed a distinction between stage-1 inhibitors, acting extracellularly, and stage-2 inhibitors, acting intracellularly (Ramel et al. 1986).

The detailed classification of mechanisms of inhibitors of mutagenesis and carcinogenesis reported in Table 1 revises and updates previous proposals (De Flora 1987, 1990, 1994, 1997; De Flora and Ramel 1988; De Flora et al. 1991, 1993, 1995a). A distinction is made between inhibitors of mutation and cancer initiation, acting either extracellularly or intracellularly, inhibitors of tumour promotion, and inhibitors of tumour progression. These mechanisms cover both inhibition and reversal of carcinogenesis, thereby fitting the previously reported definition of chemoprevention (Kelloff et al. 1994). In addition, inhibition of invasion and metastasis is also reported in Table 1. Although this objective falls within tertiary prevention rather than within chemoprevention, it is of interest to note how certain mechanisms are repetitive even in advanced stages of the carcinogenesis process.

The sequence of events occurring in the carcinogenesis process should not be oversimplified by any rigid classification into definite steps involved in the initiation-promotion-progression operative scheme (De Flora and Ramel 1988). Multiple genetic events occur along all stages of carcinogenesis (Fearon and Vogelstein 1990), and carcinogenesis has been alternatively viewed as a continuum of mutagenic and mitogenic events (Boone et al. 1992). Classifi-

Table 1. Classification of mechanisms of inhibitors of mutagenesis and carcinogenesis. (Modified from De Flora 1997)

---

1. Extracellular mechanisms
   1.1 Inhibition of uptake of mutagens/carcinogens
      1.1.1 Inhibition of penetration
      1.1.2 Removal from the organism
   1.2 Inhibition of the endogenous formation of mutagens and carcinogens
      1.2.1 Inhibition of nitrosation
      1.2.2 Modification of the intestinal microbial flora
   1.3 Complexation, dilution and/or deactivation of mutagens/carcinogens
      1.3.1 By physical or mechanical means
      1.3.2 By chemical reaction or enzyme-catalyzed reaction
   1.4 Favouring absorption of protective agents
2. Inhibition of mutation and cancer initiation by cellular mechanisms
   2.1 Stimulation of trapping and detoxification in nontarget cells
   2.2 Modification of transmembrane transport
      2.2.1 Inhibition of cellular uptake
      2.2.2 Stimulation of extrusion outside cells
   2.3 Modulation of metabolism
      2.3.1 Inhibition of activation of promutagens/procarcinogens by phase I enzymes
      2.3.2 Induction of phase I detoxification and phase II conjugation pathways, or acceleration of decomposition of reactive metabolites
      2.3.3 Stimulation of activation, coordinated with detoxification and trapping of reactive metabolites
   2.4 Blocking or competition
      2.4.1 Trapping of electrophiles by either chemical reaction or enzyme-catalyzed conjugation
      2.4.2 Antioxidant activity and scavenging of reactive oxygen species
      2.4.3 Protection of DNA nucleophilic sites
   2.5 Inhibition of cell replication
   2.6 Modulation of DNA metabolism and repair
      2.6.1 Increase of fidelity of DNA replication and repair
      2.6.2 Stimulation of repair and/or reversion of DNA damage
      2.6.3 Inhibition of error-prone repair
      2.6.4 Correction of hypomethylation
   2.7 Control of gene expression
      2.7.1 Inhibition of oncogene expression
      2.7.2 Inhibition of oncogene sequences
         2.7.2.1 Inhibition of translation directed at oncogene mRNA
         2.7.2.2 Inhibition of transcription of specific DNA sequences
         2.7.2.3 Site-specific DNA binding
      2.7.3 Neutralization of oncogene products
      2.7.4 Replacement of deleted tumour suppressor genes
      2.7.5 Killing of cells lacking tumour suppressor genes
3. Inhibition of tumour promotion
   3.1 Inhibition of genotoxic effects
   3.2 Antioxidant activity and scavenging of free radicals
   3.3 Inhibition of proteases
   3.4 Inhibition cell proliferation
   3.5 Induction of cell differentiation
   3.6 Induction of cell apoptosis
   3.7 Protection of intercellular communications
   3.8 Signal transduction modulation
   3.9 Inhibition of tumour necrosis factor α

Table 1 (continued)

4. Inhibition of tumour progression
4.1 Inhibition of genotoxic effects
4.2 Antioxidant activity and scavenging of free radicals
4.3 Inhibition of proteases
4.4 Signal transduction modulation
4.5 Effects on the hormonal status
4.6 Effects on the immune system
4.7 Inhibition of neovascularization
4.8 Physical, chemical, or biological antineoplastic activity
5. Inhibition of invasion and metastasis
5.1 Inhibition of proteases involved in basement membrane degradation and modulation of the interaction with the extracellular matrix
5.2 Induction of cell differentiation
5.3 Inhibition of neovascularization
5.4 Effect on cell-adhesion molecules
5.5 Antioxidant activity
5.6 Signal transduction modulation
5.7 Activation of antimetastasis genes

cations of mechanisms based on this concept have been also proposed (Kelloff and Boone 1994; Kelloff et al. 1994, 1996; Greenwald et al. 1995). The cascade of mechanisms shown in Table 1 should be interpreted in a flexible way, since several mechanisms are strictly interconnected or partially overlapping and important mechanisms, such as inhibition of genotoxic effects, antioxidant activity and scavening of free radicals, inhibition of cell proliferation, induction of cell differentiation, and signal transduction modulation, are reiterated several times in different phases of the process. Some mechanisms, such as "antioxidant activity and scavening of reactive oxygen species", are rather generic, and can be further subdivided according to the particular mode of action of each agent.

Multiple Mechanisms of Chemopreventive Agents

Table 1 shows a schema of individual mechanisms by which inhibitors can exert their protective effects. Actually, it is rather uncommon for a given agent to be so specialized as to intervene at one level only. Most chemopreventive agents are known or thought to work through multiple mechanisms because of the involvement of pleiotropic properties. Unfortunately, some of these properties may be negative and lead to adverse effects in term of toxicity, or even of genotoxicity and carcinogenicity, often depending on doses, route of administration, schedule of exposure to carcinogenes and chemopreventive agents, for example (De Flora and Ramel 1988). Even physiological mechanisms are generally double-edged swords, although for some of them the protective role is dominant. In principle, chemopreventive agents with multiple mechanisms of action are expected to be more effective and to have a broader spectrum of protective activity against different carcinogens and in various exposure conditions.

Examples of chemopreventive agents possessing different protective mechanisms are given below. The list, which is far from being exhaustive, includes 18 compounds, most of which are considered to be among the most promising cancer chemopreventive agents (Kelloff and Boone 1994). For the sake of simplicity, the mechanisms reported for each of them use the same wording as in the classification of individual mechanisms (Table 1). More details on the precise mechanisms for each compound can be inferred from the references cited. The numerical codes in square brackets correspond to the identification numbers of the mechanisms shown in Table 1. Because it is such a vast literature, only a limited number of references are given for each compound, and priority was given to review articles, in which further details and references can be found.

N-Acetylcysteine (NAC) and Other Thiols

Inhibition of nitrosation [1.2.1]; modification of the intestinal microbial flora [1.2.2]; stimulation of trapping and detoxification in nontarget cells [2.1]; stimulation of activation, coordinated with detoxification and trapping of reactive metabolites [2.3.3]; trapping of electrophiles [2.4.1]; antioxidant activity and scavenging of reactive oxygen species [2.4.2, 3.2, 4.2, 5.5]; stimulation of repair and/or reversion of DNA damage [2.6.2]; correction of hypomethylation [2.6.4]; inhibition of genotoxic effects [3.1, 4.1]; signal transduction modulation [3.8, 4.4, 5.6]; inhibition of neovascularization [4.7, 5.3]; inhibition of proteases involved is basement membrane degradation and modulation of the interaction with the extracellular matrix [5.1] (Bergelson et al. 1994; De Flora et al. 1995a,b; van Zandwijk 1995; Albini et al. 1995; Giunciuglio et al. 1996; Kelloff et al. 1996; Lertratanangkoon et al. 1996).

Calcium

Inhibition of penetration [1.1.1]; modification of the intestinal microbial flora [1.2.2]; complexation of mutagens/carcinogens [1.3]; inhibition of cellular uptake [2.2.1]; inhibition of cell replication [2.5, 3.4]; inhibition of oncogene expression [2.7.1]; inhibition of genotoxic effects [3.1, 4.1]; induction of cell differentiation [3.5, 5.2] (Wargovich et al. 1983; De Flora and Ramel 1988; De Flora et al. 1991, 1993; Govers et al. 1994; Kelloff and Boone 1994; Greenwald et al. 1995; Lipkin and Newmark 1995).

β-Carotene

Inhibition of activation of promutagens/procarcinogens by phase I enzymes [2.3.1]; antioxidant activity and scavening of reactive oxygen species [2.4.2, 3.2, 4.2, 5.5]; inhibition of cell replication [2.5; 3.4]; inhibition of genotoxic effects [3.1, 4.1]; protection of intercellular communications [3.7] (Krinski 1993; De Flora et al. 1993; Kelloff and Boone 1994; Nishino 1995; Kelloff et al. 1996).

Chlorophyllin and Haemin

Inhibition of activation of promutagens/procarcinogens by phase I enzymes [2.3.1]; trapping of electrophiles [2.4.1]; inhibition of genotoxic effects [3.1; 4.1] (Hartman and Shankel 1990; Tachino et al. 1994; Arimoto et al. 1995).

Dehydroepiandrosterone (DHEA) and Analogues

Inhibition of activation of promutagens/procarcinogens by phase I enzymes [2.3.1]; inhibition of cell replication [2.5, 3.4]; inhibition of genotoxic effects [3.1, 4.1]; signal transduction modulation [3.8, 4.4, 5.6] (Feo et al. 1984; Greenwald et al. 1995; Schwartz and Pashko 1995; Kelloff et al. 1996).

Flavonoids

Inhibition of activation of promutagens/procarcinogens by phase I enzymes [2.3.1]; trapping of electrophiles [2.4.1]; inhibition of genotoxic effects [3.1, 4.1]; induction of cell apoptosis [3.6]; signal transduction modulation [3.8, 4.4, 5.6] (De Flora and Ramel 1988; Weinstein 1988; De Flora et al. 1991; Greenwald et al. 1995; Kelloff et al. 1996; Lepley et al. 1996).

Indoles

Inhibition of activation of promutagens/procarcinogens by phase I enzymes [2.3.1]; induction of phase I detoxification and phase II conjugation pathways, or acceleration of decomposition of reactive metabolites [2.3.2]; stimulation of activation, coordinated with detoxification and trapping of reactive metabolites [2.3.3]; inhibition of genotoxic effects [3.1, 4.1] (Fong et al. 1990; De Flora et al. 1991; Takahashi et al. 1995).

Isothiocyanates

Inhibition of activation of promutagens/procarcinogens by phase I enzymes [2.3.1]; induction of phase I detoxification and phase II conjugation pathways [2.3.2]; inhibition of cell replication [2.5, 3.4]; inhibition of genotoxic effects [3.1, 4.1] (Wattenberg 1977; De Flora et al. 1991; Stoner et al. 1991; Hecht 1995; Conaway et al. 1996; Yu et al. 1996).

Nonsteroidal Anti-Inflammatory Drugs (NSAIDS)

Antioxidant activity and scavenging of reactive oxygen species [2.4.2, 3.2, 4.2, 5.5]; inhibition of cell replication [2.5, 3.4]; inhibition of genotoxic effects [3.1, 4.1]; signal transduction modulation [3.8, 4.4, 5.6] (Greenwald et al. 1995; Kelloff et al. 1996).

Oltipraz and Other Dithiolthiones

Inhibition of activation of promutagens/procarcinogens by phase I enzymes [2.3.1]; induction of phase I detoxification and phase II conjugation pathways [2.3.2]; trapping of electrophiles [2.4.1]; inhibition of genotoxic effects [3.1, 4.1] (Wattenberg and Bueding 1986; Kensler et al. 1987; Egner et al. 1994; Kensler and Helzlsouer 1995).

Phenols (Natural and Synthetic)

Inhibition of nitrosation [1.2.1]; inhibition of activation of promutagens/procarcinogens by phase I enzymes [2.3.1]; induction of phase I detoxification and phase II conjugation pathways [2.3.2]; trapping of electrophiles [2.4.1]; antioxidant activity and scavenging of reactive oxygen species [2.4.2, 3.2, 4.2, 5.5]; inhibition of genotoxic effects [3.1, 4.1]; induction of apoptosis [3.6]; signal transduction modulation [3.8, 4.4, 5.6]; inhibition of proteases involved in basement membrane degradation and modulation of the interaction with the extracellular matrix [5.1] (Bartsch et al. 1988; Huang et al. 1991; De Flora et al. 1991; Stoner and Mukhtar 1995; Suganuma et al. 1996; Kelloff et al. 1996; Jiang et al. 1996; Stetler-Stevenson et al. 1996).

Protease Inhibitors

Antioxidant activity and scavenging of reactive oxygen species [2.4.2, 3.2, 4.2, 5.5]; inhibition of error-prone DNA repair [2.6.3]; inhibition of oncogene expression [2.7.1]; inhibition of genotoxic effects [3.1, 4.1]; inhibition of proteases [3.3, 4.3]; inhibition of proteases involved in basement membrane de-

gradation and modulation of the interaction with the extracellular matrix
[5.1] (De Flora et al. 1991; Kennedy 1993; Greenwald et al. 1995; Kelloff et al.
1996).

Selenium (Inorganic and Organic Compounds)

Antioxidant activity and scavenging of reactive oxygen species [2.4.2, 3.2,
4.2, 5.5]; inhibition of cell replication [2.5, 3.4]; inhibition of genotoxic effects [3.1, 4.1]; effects on the immune system [4.6] (Shamberger 1986; De
Flora et al. 1991; Ip and Ganther 1992; Greenwald et al. 1995; El-Bayoumi et
al. 1995; Kelloff et al. 1996).

Tamoxifen

Antioxidant activity and scavenging of reactive oxygen species [2.4.2, 3.2,
4.2, 5.5]; inhibition of cell replication [2.5, 3.4]; inhibition of genotoxic effects [3.1, 4.1]; induction of cell apoptosis [3.6]; signal transduction modulation [3.8, 4.4, 5.6]; inhibition of tumour necrosis factor α [3.9]; effects on the
hormonal status [4.5]; inhibition of neovascularization [4.7, 5.3] (Jordan and
Murphy 1990; Nayfield et al. 1991; Kelloff and Boone 1994; Kelloff et al. 1996;
Suganuma et al. 1996; IARC 1996).

Vitamin A (Retinol) and Analogues (Retinoids)

Protection of DNA nucleophilic sites [2.4.3]; inhibition of cell replication
[2.5, 3.4]; inhibition of oncogene expression [2.7.1]; inhibition of genotoxic
effects [3.1, 4.1]; induction of cell differentiation [3.5, 5.2]; induction of cell
apoptosis [3.6]; protection of intercellular communications [3.7]; signal transduction modulation [3.8, 4.4, 5.6]; effects on the immune system [4.6]; inhibition of neovascularization [4.7, 5.3]; inhibition of proteases involved in
basement membrane degradation and modulation of the interaction with the
extracellular matrix [5.1] (Shamberger 1986; De Flora and Ramel 1988,
Greenwald et al. 1995; Lippman et al. 1995; Kelloff et al. 1996).

Vitamin C (Ascorbic-Acid)

Inhibition of nitrosation [1.2.1]; antioxidant activity and scavenging of reactive oxygen species [2.4.2, 3.2, 4.2, 5.5]; inhibition of genotoxic effects [3.1,
4.1] (Shamberger 1986; Bartsch et al. 1988; De Flora et al. 1991).

Vitamin D₃ (cholecalciferol) and Analogues (Deltanoids)

Favouring absorption of protective agents [1.4]; inhibition of cell replication [2.5, 3.4]; inhibition of genotoxic effects [3.1, 4.1]; induction of cell differentiation [3.5, 5.2] (Kelloff and Boone 1994; Greenwald et al. 1995; Norman 1995).

Vitamin E (α-Tocopherol)

Inhibition of nitrosation [1.2.1]; antioxidant activity and scavenging of reactive oxygen species [2.4.2, 3.2, 4.2, 5.5]; inhibition of genotoxic effects [3.1, 4.1]; effects on the immune system [4.6] (Shamberger 1986; Bartsch et al. 1988; De Flora et al. 1991; Kelloff et al. 1996).

Requirements of Chemopreventive Agents

The practical application of chemopreventive agents should take into account some basic requirements, such as (a) cost, as related to cost-benefit analyses; (b) practically of use, such as availability, stability, convenience of the administration route and schedule; (c) efficacy; and (d) safety (De Flora et al. 1996 a). It is evident that the maximum of technically available efficacy is needed for the treatment of cancer patients, even though the cost may be high, practicality of use may be poor, and severe side effects may often occur. On the other hand, tolerability is the main prerequisite in public health interventions addressed to healthy subjects in the population. For the time being, this approach of primary prevention may be restricted to dietary education of the public. The lack of side-effects, evaluated on the base of risk-benefit analyses, may be less stringent when chemoprevention is extended to the use of pharmacological agents and is either applied in a primary prevention setting but in high-risk individuals (targeted chemoprevention) or in a secondary prevention setting with the aim of preventing second primaries or achieving regression of premalignant lesions.

Certainly, more basic research is still needed for a broader application of chemoprevention. It is a lucky coincidence, however, that some of the most promising chemopreventive agents (e. g., NSAIDs, NAC, or vitamins) already find extensive use in the population for various therapeutic purposes. Other agents are not only available as natural food components or dietary supplements, but are also commonly used for food preservation, especially because of their antioxidant activity. There is also need for a further advancement in the cultural preparation of the medical class and health personnel. Dietary and pharmacological interventions aimed at certain altered conditions, such as high blood pressure or dyslipidosis, which up to a few years ago were quite controversial, proved to be successful and are now widely accepted as important prevention measures in the control of cardiovascular diseases.

Cancer chemoprevention is still a young discipline, but the continuously growing interest of the scientific community is documented by the higher and higher proportion of scientific articles and symposia dealing with basic concepts, experimental studies, and application in clinical trials of this strategy for cancer prevention.

References

Albini A, D'Agostini F, Giunciuglio D, Paglieri I, Balansky R, De Flora S (1995) Inhibition of invasion, gelatinase activity, tumor take and metastasis of malignant cells by N-acetylcysteine. Int J Cancer 61:121–129

Arimoto S, Kan-yama K, Rai H, Hayatsu H (1995) Inhibitory effect of hemin, clorophyllin and related pyrrole pigments on the mutagenicity of benzo[a]pyrene and its metabolites. Mutat Res 345:127–135

Bartsch H, Ohshima H, Pignatelli B (1988) Inhibitors of endogenous nitrosation. Mechanisms and implications in human cancer prevention. Mutat Res 202:307–324

Bergelson S, Pinkus R, Daniel V (1994) Intracellular glutathione levels regulate fos/jun induction and activation of glutathione S-transferase gene expression. Cancer Res 54:36–40

Bertram JS, Kolonel LN, Meyskens FL Jr (1987) Rationale and strategies for chemoprevention of cancer in humans. Cancer Res 47:3012–3031

Boone CW, Kelloff GJ, Steele VE (1992) Natural history of intraepithelial neoplasia in humans with implications for cancer chemopreventive strategy. Cancer Res 52:1651–1659

Conaway CC, Jiao D, Chung FL (1996) Inhibition of rat liver cytochrome P450 isozymes by isothiocyanates and their conjugates: a structure-activity relationship study. Carcinogenesis 17:2423–2427

De Flora S (1987) Proposed classification of inhibitors of mutagenesis and carcinogenesis according to their mechanisms (abstract). 2nd International Conference on Anticarcinogenesis and Radiation Protection, Gaithersburg, Md, 8–12 March 1987

De Flora S (1990) Mechanisms of inhibitors of genotoxicity. Relevance in preventive medicine. In: Mendelsohn ML, Albertini RJ (eds) Mutation and the environment, part E. Wiley-Liss, New York, pp 307–318

De Flora S (1994) Cancer prevention strategies and mechanisms of chemopreventive agents. Eur J Cancer Prev 3:364–366

De Flora S (1998) Mechanisms of inhibitors of mutagenesis and carcinogenesis. Mutat Res 402:151–158

De Flora S, Ramel C (1988) Mechanisms of inhibitors of mutagenesis and carcinogenesis. Classification and overview. Mutat Res 202:285–306

De Flora S, Zanacchi P, Izzotti A, Hayatsu H (1991) Mechanisms of food-borne inhibitors of genotoxicity relevant to cancer prevention. In: Hayatsu H (ed) Mutagens in food. Detection and prevention. CRC Press, Boca Raton, Fl, pp 157–180

De Flora S, Bronzetti G, Sobels FH (eds) (1992) Assessment of antimutagenicity and anticarcinogenicity. End-points and systems. Mutat Res 267:153–295

De Flora S, Izzotti A, Bennicelli C (1993) Mechanisms if antimutagenesis and anticarcinogenesis. Role in primary prevention. In: Bronzetti G, Hayatsu H, De Flora S, Waters MD, Shankel DM (eds) Antimutagenesis and anticarcinogenesis mechanisms, vol III. Plenum Press, New York, pp 1–16

De Flora S, Balansky R, Bennicelli C, Camoirano A, D'Agostini F, Izzotti A, Cesarone CF (1995a) Mechanisms of anticarcinogenesis: the example of N-acetylcysteine. In: Ioannides C, Lewis DFV (eds) Drugs, diet and disease, vol 1: Mechanistic approaches to cancer. Ellis Horwood, Hemel Hempstead, UK, pp 151–203

De Flora S, Cesarone CF, Balansky RM, Albini A, D'Agostini F, Bennicelli C, Bagnasco M, Camoirano A, Scatolini L, Rovida A, Izzotti A (1995b) Chemopreventive properties and mechanisms of *N*-acetylcysteine. The experimental background. J Cell Biochem 58 [Suppl 22]:33–41

De Flora S, Balansky R, Scatolini L, Di Marco C, Gasparini L, Orlando M, Izzotti A (1996a) Adducts to nuclear DNA and mitochondrial DNA as biomarkers in chemoprevention. In: Stewart BW, McGregor D, Kleihues P (eds) Principles of chemoprevention. (IARC scientific publication no 139) International Agency for Research on Cancer, Lyon, pp 291–301

De Flora S, Izzotti A, Randerath K, Randerath E, Bartsch H, Nair J, Balansky R, van Schooten F, Degan P, Fronza G, Walsh D, Lewtas J (1996b) DNA adducts and chronic degenerative diseases. Pathogenetic relevance and implications in preventive medicine. Mutat Res 366:197–238

Egner PA, Kensler TW, Prestera T, Talalay P, Libby AH, Curphey TJ (1994) Regulation of phase 2 enzyme induction by otipraz and other dithiolethiones. Carcinogenesis 15:177–181

El-Bayoumy K, Upadhyaya P, Chae Y-H, Sohn O-S, Rao CV, Fiala E, Reddy BS (1995) Chemoprevention of cancer by organoselenium compounds. J Cell Biochem Suppl 22:92–100

Fearon ER, Vogelstein B (1990) A genetic model for colorectal tumorigenesis. Cell 61:759–767

Feo F, Pirisi L, Pascale R, Daino L, Frassetto S, Garcea R, Gaspa L (1984) Modulatory effect of glucose-6-phosphate dehydrogenase deficiency on benzo(*a*)pyrene toxicity and transforming activity for in vitro-cultured human skin fibroblasts. Cancer Res 44:3419–3425

Fong AT, Swanson HI, Dashwood RH, Williams DE, Hendricks JD, Bailey GS (1990) Mechanisms of anti-carcinogenesis by indole-3-carbinol: studies of enzyme induction, electrophile-scavenging, and inhibition of aflatoxin B_1 activation. Biochem Pharmacol 39:19–26

Giunciuglio D, Cai T, Masiello L, De Flora S, Albini A (1996) *N*-Acetylcysteine. A possible inhibitor of tumor angiogenesis (abstract). Presented at the Meeting on Oxidative Stress and Redox Regulation, Paris, France, 21–24 May 1996

Govers MJAP, Termont DSML, van der Meer R (1994) Mechanisms of the antiproliferative effect of milk mineral and other calcium supplements on colonic epithelium. Cancer Res 54:95–100

Greenwald P, Kelloff GJ, Boone CW, McDonald SS (1995) Genetic and cellular changes in colorectal cancer: proposed targets of chemopreventive agents. Cancer Epidemiol Biomarkers Prev 4:691–702

Hartman PE, Shankel DM (1990) Antimutagens anticarcinogens: a survey of putative interceptor molecules. Environ Mol Mutagen 15:145–182

Hecht SS (1995) Chemoprevention by isothiocyanates. J Cell Biochem Suppl 22:195–209

Huang T-S, Lee S-C, Lin J-K (1991) Suppression of c-Jun/AP-1 activation by an inhibitor of tumor promotion in mouse fibroblast cells. Proc Natl Acad Sci USA 88:5292–5296

International Agency for Research on Cancer (1996) Some pharmaceutical drugs. IARC Monogr Eval Carcinog Risks Hum 66:253–365

Ip C, Ganther HE (1992) Relationship between the chemical form of selenium and anticarcinogenic activity. In: Wattenberg, Lipkin M, Boone CW, Kelloff GJ (eds) Cancer chemoprevention. CRC Press, Boca Raton, Fl, pp 479–488

Jiang M-C, Yang-Yen H-F, Jong-Young Yen J, Lin J-K (1996) Curcumin induces apoptosis in immortalized NIH 3T3 and malignant cancer cell lines. Nutr Cancer 26:111–120

Jordan VC, Murphy CS (1990) Endocrine pharmacology of antiestrogens as antitumor agents. Endocr Rev 11:578–610

Kada T, Inoue T, Namiki N (1982) Environmental desmutagens and antimutagens. In: Klekowski EJ (ed) Environmental mutagenesis and plant biology. Praeger, New York, pp 137–151

Kelloff GJ, Boone CW (eds) (1994) Cancer chemopreventive agents. Drug development status and future prospects. J Cell Biochem Suppl 20:1–303

Kelloff GJ, Boone CW, Steele VE, Crowell JA, Lubet R, Sigman CC (1994) Progress in cancer chemoprevention: perspectives on agent selection and short-term clinical intervention trials. Cancer Res 54 [Suppl]:2015s–2024s

Kelloff GJ, Boone CW, Steele VE, Crowell JA, Lubet RA, Greenwald P, Hawk ET, Fay JR, Sigman CC (1996) Mechanistic considerations in the evaluation of chemopreventive data.

In: Stewart BW, McGregor D, Kleihues P (eds) Principles of chemoprevention. (IARC scientific publication no 139). International Agency for Research on Cancer, Lyon, pp 203–219

Kennedy AR (1993) Overview: anticarcinogenic activity of protease inhibitors. In: Troll W, Kennedy AR (eds) Protease inhibitors as cancer chemopreventive agents. Plenum, New York, pp 9–64

Kensler TW, Helzlsouer KJ (1995) Oltipraz: clinical opportunities for cancer chemoprevention. J Cell Biochem Suppl 22:101–107

Kensler TW, Egner PA, Dolan PM, Groopman JD, Roebuck BD (1987) Mechanism of protection against aflatoxin tumorigenicity in rats fed 5-(2-pyrazinyl)-4-methyl-1,2-dithiol-3-thione (oltipraz) and related 1,2-dithiol-3-thione and 1,2-dithiol-3-ones. Cancer Res 47:4271–4277

Krinsky NI (1993) Actions of carotenoids in biological systems. Annu Rev Nutr 13:561–587

Last JM (1986) Scope and methods of prevention. In: Last JM, Chin J, Fielding JE, Frank AL, Lashof JC, Wallace RB (eds) Maxcy-Rosenau. Public health and preventive medicine. Appleton-Century-Crofts, Norwalk, Ct, pp 3–7

Lepley DM, Li B, Birt DF, Pelling JC (1996) The chemopreventive flavonoid apigenin induces G_2/M arrest in keratinocytes. Carcinogenesis 17:2367–2375

Lertratanangkoon K, Orkiszewski RS, Scimeca JM (1996) Methyl-donors deficiency due to chemically induced glutathione depletion. Cancer Res 56:995–1005

Lipkin M, Newmark H (1995) Calcium and the prevention of colon cancer. J Cell Biochem Suppl 22:65–73

Lippman SM, Heyman RA, Kurie JM, Benner SE, Hong WK (1995) Retinoids and chemoprevention: clinical and basic studies. J Cell Biochem Suppl 22:1–10

Morse MA, Stoner GD (1993) Cancer chemoprevention: principles and prospects. Carcinogenesis 14:1737–1746

Nayfield SG, Karp JE, Ford LG, Dorr FA, Kramer BS (1991) Potential role of tamoxifen in prevention of breast cancer. J Natl Cancer Inst 83:1450–1459

Nishino H (1995) Cancer chemoprevention by natural carotenoids and their related compounds. J Cell Biochem Suppl 22:231–235

Norman AW (1995) The vitamin D endocrine system: manipulation of structure-function relationships to provide opportunities for development of new cancer chemopreventive and immunosuppresive agents. J Cell Biochem Suppl 22:218–225

Ramel C, Alekperov UK, Ames BN, Kada T, Wattenberg LW (1986) Inhibitors of mutagenesis and their relevance to carcinogenesis. Mutat Res 168:47–65

Schwartz AG, Pashko LL (1995) Cancer prevention with dehydroepiandrosterone and non-androgenic structural analogs. J Cell Biochem Suppl 22:210–217

Shamberger RJ (1986) Chemoprevention of cancer. In: Reddy BS, Cohen LA (eds) Diet, nutrition, and cancer: a critical evaluation, vol II: Micronutrients, nonnutritive dietary factors, and cancer. CRC Press, Boca Raton, Fl, pp 43–62

Sporn MB, Newton DL (1979) Chemoprevention of cancer with retinoids. Fed Proc 38:2528–2534

Stetler-Stevenson WG, Hewitt R, Corcoran M (1996) Matrix metalloproteinases and tumor invasion: from correlation and causality to the clinic. Semin Cancer Biol 7:147–154

Stoner GD; Mukthar H (1995) Polyphenols as cancer chemopreventive agents. J Cell Biochem Suppl 22:169–180

Stoner GD, Morrissey D, Heur Y-H, Daniel E, Galati A, Wagner SA (1991) Inhibitory effects of phenethyl isothiocyanate on *N*-nitrosobenzylmethylamine carcinogenesis in the rat esophagus. Cancer Res 51:2063–2068

Suganuma M, Okabe S, Sueoka E, Iida N, Komori A, Kim S-J, Fujiki H (1996) A new process of cancer prevention mediated through inhibition of tumor necrosis factor α expression. Cancer Res 56:3711–3715

Tachino N, Guo D, Dashwood WM, Yamane S, Larsen R, Dashwood RH (1994) Mechanisms of the in vitro anti-mutagenic action of chlorophyllin against benzo[*a*]pyrene: studies of enzyme inhibition, molecular complex formation, and degradation of the ultimate carcinogen. Mutat Res 308:191–203

Takahashi N, Dashwood RH, Bjeldanes LF, Bailey GS, Williams DE (1995) Regulation of hepatic CYP 1 A 1 by indol-3-carbinol: transient induction with continuous feeding in rainbow trout. Food Chem Toxicol 33:111–120

Trosko J, Chang C (1980) An integrative hypothesis linking cancer, diabetes, and atherosclerosis: The role of mutations and epigenetic changes. Med Hypotheses 6:455–468

van Zandwijk N (1995) N-Acetylcysteine (NAC) and glutathione (GSH): antioxidant and chemopreventive properties, with special reference to lung cancer. J Cell Biochem Suppl 22:24–32

Wargovich MJ, Eng VWS, Newmark HL, Bruce WR (1983) Calcium ameliorates the toxic effect of deoxycholic acid on colonic epithelium. Carcinogenesis 4:1205–1207

Wattenberg LW (1977) Inhibition of carcinogenic effects of polycyclic hydrocarbons by benzyl isothiocyanate and related compounds. J Natl Cancer Inst 58:395–398

Wattenberg LW (1981) Inhibitors of chemical carcinogens. In: Burchenal JH, Oettgen HF (eds) Cancer: achievements, challenges and prospects for the 1980 s. Grune and Stratton, New York, pp 517–540

Wattenberg LW, Bueding E (1986) Inhibitory effects of 5-(2-pyranizyl)-4-methyl-1,2-dithiol-3-thione (oltipraz) on carcinogenesis induced by benzo[a]pyrene, diethylnitrosamine and uracil mustard. Carcinogenesis 7:1379–1381

Weinstein IB (1988) Strategies for inhibiting multistage carcinogenesis based on signal transduction pathways. Mutat Res 202:413–420

Yu R, Jiao J-J, Duh J-L, Tan T-H, Tony Kong A-N (1996) Phenethyl isothiocyanate, a natural chemopreventive agent, activates c-Jun N-terminal kinase 1. Cancer Res 56:2954–2955

Metabolic Targets of Cancer Chemoprevention: Interruption of Tumor Development by Inhibitors of Arachidonic Acid Metabolism

F. Marks, G. Fürstenberger, and K. Müller-Decker

Tumor Cell Regulation, Department B 0500, German Cancer Research Center, D-69120 Heidelberg, Germany

Abstract

Tumor promotion is understood as a process that favors the clonal outgrowth of single mutated (initiated) cells to premalignant lesions through co-mitogenic and anti-apoptotic effects. This process can be evoked by repeated induction of a regenerative tissue response as achieved either by irritation and wounding or by agents (tumor promoters) that interact with the corresponding pathways of cellular signaling. Metabolic processes regulated by such pathways and essential for tumor development are potential targets of cancer chemoprevention. Examples are provided by the expression of ornithine decarboxylase and the activation of eicosanoid formation from arachidonic acid. Arachidonic acid metabolism is a particularly attractive and important target of chemopreventive measures. Its induction is a characteristic response to tissue damage and irritation and an apparently critical event in epithelial tumor promotion. Inhibitors of eicosanoid formation, such as nonsteroidal anti-inflammatory drugs, rank among the most powerful chemopreventive agents in animal models and have been shown to halve the incidence of colorectal cancer in man. Recently, the role of cyclooxygenase-2 (COX-2)-catalyzed prostaglandin synthesis has been the subject of much attention. COX-2 is a typical 'emergency enzyme', since in most tissues it is transiently induced only in the course of repair and defense reactions. In epithelial neoplasia, i.e. in skin and colorectal tumors, the enzyme is constitutively overexpressed along different molecular pathways, and it seems to be critically involved in tumor promotion. Consequently, specific COX-2 inhibitors have been shown to exhibit considerable cancer chemopreventive potential. The putative role of other pathways of arachidonic acid metabolism in tumor promotion and malignant progression is presently under investigation.

Introduction

Cancer is the result of an irregular developmental process, which is based on a sequential accumulation of gene mutations. Thus, chemoprevention, i.e. the

Recent Results in Cancer Research, Vol. 151
Senn/Costa/Jordan (Eds.): Chemoprevention of Cancer
© Springer-Verlag Berlin · Heidelberg 1999

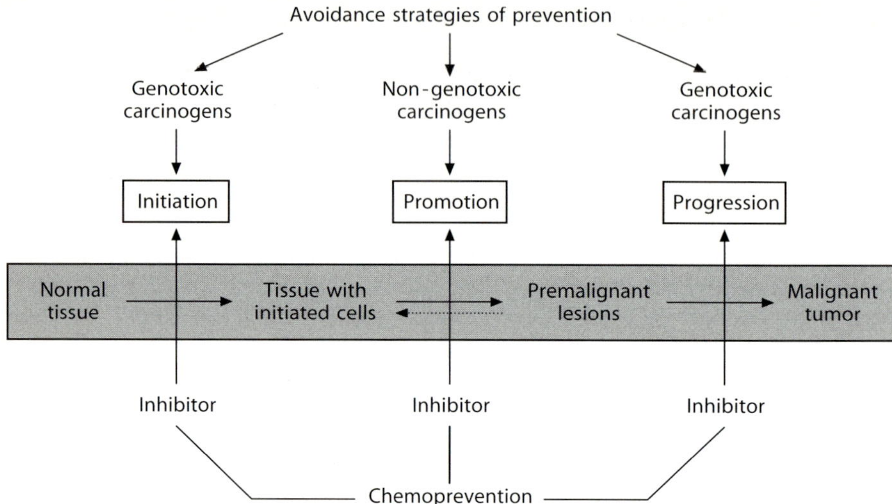

Fig. 1. Strategies of cancer prevention. A malignant tumor results from a developmental process that is due to a series of genetic alterations caused by environmental and endogenous genotoxic factors. Especially in the premalignant phase, this process is promoted by non-genotoxic carcinogens. While avoidance strategies of cancer prevention aim at an elimination of genotoxic and non-genotoxic carcinogens, the major targets of chemoprevention are the metabolic processes involved in the different stages of tumor development

prevention of cancer by drugs or nutrients, has two major goals: (1) to interfere with the genotoxic insults, thereby preventing neoplastic development at the roots; and (2) to interfere with mechanisms of neoplastic progression, thus bringing cancer development to a halt at a premalignant stage.

While the great majority of the gene mutations evoking neoplastic growth are thought to be due to environmental factors with which contact could generally be avoided, neoplastic progression seems to proceed mainly along endogenous pathways that are targets of enzyme inhibitors, antimetabolites, and related drugs. These endogenous mechanisms of tumor development may be considered, therefore, to provide the targets proper of cancer chemoprevention (Fig. 1).

Tumor Promotion as a Potential Target of Chemoprevention

The genetic alterations causing neoplastic progression include the activation of proto-oncogenes and the inhibition or deletion of so-called suppressor genes. It is generally assumed that neoplastic development starts with the mutation of one such gene in a single cell. This process is traditionally called initiation.

The accumulation of genetic defects correlates with distinct clinical symptoms, such as dysplastic growth, benign tumor, carcinoma in situ, and destructive metastasizing cancer. While genetic and morphological analysis of human neoplasia have impressively demonstrated the gradual development of cancer (Brown et al. 1994; Kinzler and Vogelstein 1996), our knowledge of the underlying mechanisms is based mainly on animal experiments, which allow dissection of tumorigenesis into distinct stages. Classical models of multistage carcinogenesis are provided by skin cancer of mice (DiGiovanni 1992; Marks and Fürstenberger 1995) and liver cancer of rats (Schwarz 1995). In both models the initial oncogenic mutation has been found to be irreversible. However, this situation does not mean that a tumor will develop inevitably. Indeed, initiated cells can remain in the tissue as 'dormant tumor cells' for any period of time. This is because of the extremely low probability that the additional genetic changes required for neoplastic progression occur in a particular single cell. The probability increases, however, as the initiated cell expands into a clone. Clonal expansion is dramatically accelerated by so-called tumor-promoting factors.

Such factors are widespread in our environment and include industrial chemicals, nutrients, tobacco smoke, alcohol, viruses, and UV irradiation. The great majority of so-called non-genotoxic carcinogens (Grasso et al. 1991; Shaw and Jones 1994) can be looked on as tumor promoters. To the best of our knowledge, tumor promotion depends on the repeated induction of metabolic changes, rather than on gene mutations. On the other hand, these metabolic changes may give rise to an accumulation of genotoxic metabolites, which then may promote further oncogenic mutations and, thus, progression towards malignancy. This means it may be that neither premalignant nor malignant lesions can develop without promotion. Therefore, the metabolic processes involved in tumor promotion present particularly attractive targets of cancer chemoprevention. Moreover, a chemopreventive approach aiming at interruption of tumor development rather than complete eradication of tumor cells does not depend on progress in approaches that have still to be developed, such as gene therapy.

Theoretically, tumor promotion may result from a combined effect on cellular proliferation and cell death by apoptosis, terminal differentiation, or cytotoxicity. A permanent repetition of the promoting stimulus would then offer a selective advantage for initiated cells, providing they are more sensitive to mitogenic and less sensitive to inhibitory and death signals than the normal cells surrounding them.

Tissue regeneration and wound healing are processes that typically involve dramatic effects on both cell proliferation and cell differentiation/cell death. The mouse model of skin carcinogenesis has indeed provided ample evidence that tumor promotion can proceed along the pathways of tissue regeneration. Thus, the simplest way to promote skin tumorigenesis is by repeated wounding, whereas chemical skin tumor promoters evoke a pseudo-wound response, i.e. a hyperplastic and inflammatory reaction, either by unspecific irritation or by interaction with intracellular pathways that are normally involved in the processing of wound-related signals, such as cytokines and growth factors (Marks and Fürstenberger 1995).

Tumor Promotion Results from an Inadequate Stimulation of Signaling Cascades

Tumor promotion by the repeated disturbance of intracellular signaling is best exemplified by the action of the phorbol ester TPA. This extremly active skin tumor promoter mimics specifically the cellular effects of the second messenger diacylglycerol (DAG). DAG is released together with inositol-1,4,5-trisphosphate from membrane phospholipids by the receptor-controlled phospholipase C isoenzymes (Fig. 2). Major targets of DAG in the cell are the protein kinases of the C class (PKC), which occupy a central position in cellular signal processing, in that they convey the signals from a large number of receptors to the cell nucleus (Marks and Gschwendt 1996). On many cell types PKC activation exerts both a mitogenic and an antiapoptotic effect: that is to say it ideally fulfills the requirements of a tumor-promoting stimulus. However, because of the multiplicity of the PKC family (including 11 isoenzymes so far), the large number of potential PKC substrate proteins, and the extraordinarily high degree of interaction of PKC with other signal-transducing factors, the molecular mechanisms underlying the role of PKC in tumor promotion are still not fully understood (Marks and Gschwendt 1995). On the other hand, numerous phorbol ester/DAG-responsive genes thought to be under the control of PKC have been identified. These genes are regulated by the AP-1 transcription factor family consisting of dimers of Jun, Fos, and ATF proteins (Karin et al. 1997). AP-1 transcription factors are targets of several signal-transducing pathways, in particular of the so-called MAP kinase cascades (Seger and Krebs 1995). This cascades represent a series of major signaling pathways leading from the cell's periphery into the nucleus (Denhardt 1996; Treisman 1996). One of the cascades seems to play a key role in tumor promotion, at least in the skin. Upon wounding, this so-called Ras/Raf/Erk cascade becomes transiently activated by growth factors such as TGFα, whereas the tumor promoter TPA makes a short cut by activating protein kinase C, which in turn stimulates the protein kinase Raf-1 (see Fig. 2; Naumann et al. 1996). As a consequence, a series of genes is activated which control cell proliferation and other processes. In addition, programmed cell death is suppressed by an activated Ras/Raf/Erk cascade (Wang et al. 1996).

Several components and target proteins of the cascade are subject to oncogenic mutation. In the mouse skin model of carcinogenesis the oncogenic activation of the *H-ras* gene appears to provide a major initiating event, which results in a *H-ras* protein that is defective in signal extinction (Balmain and Brown 1988). It is easily conceivable that initiated cells harboring a deregulated Ras/Raf/Erk cascade respond more sensitively to mitogenic and less sensitively to apoptotic signals than do normal cells. Moreover, since the biosynthesis of growth factors, such as TGFα is most probably induced along the cascade (Glick et al. 1991; Coffey et al. 1992; Klein et al. 1992), a positive autocrine feedback loop (Imamoto et al. 1991) is expected to develop in tumor cells, which results in a constitutive overexpression of TGFα and other proteins controlled by the Ras/Raf/Erk cascade (Fig. 2). In the conditions of

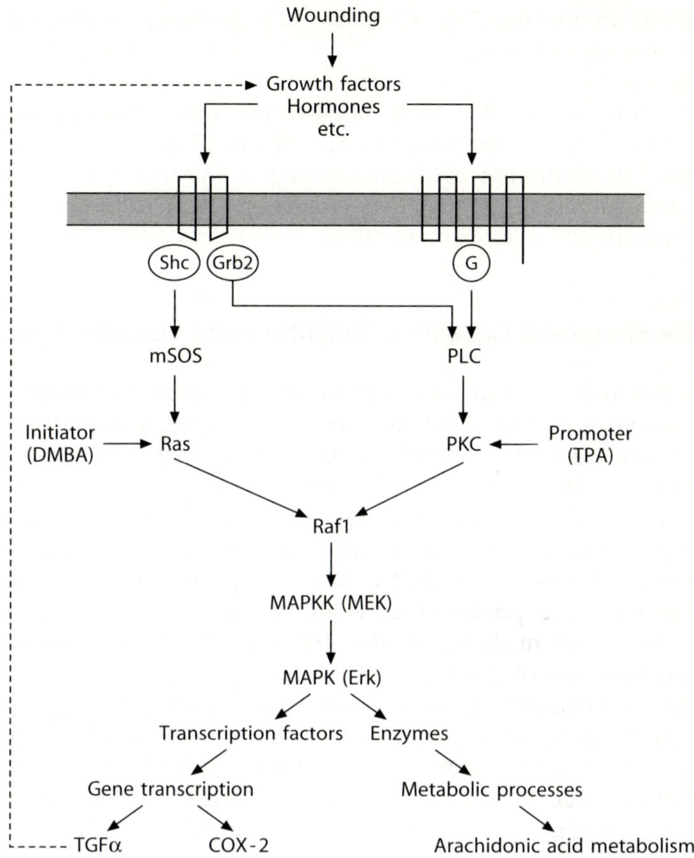

Fig. 2. Major pathways of intracellular signal transduction as targets of genotoxic and non-genotoxic carcinogens. The scheme shows a highly simplified 'switching diagram' for the biochemical device used by vertebrate cells for the processing of a wide variety of extracellular signals which – for instance when released upon wounding – regulate cell proliferation, cell differentiation and programmed cell death. Transmembrane signaling is accomplished both by dimeric receptor proteins, which upon ligand binding undergo (auto)-phosphorylation on Tyr residues (*left branch*), and by receptors consisting of seven transmembrane domains (7 TMD-R; *right branch*), which in turn activate trimeric G-proteins. The Tyr-phosphorylated receptors activate several proteins via interactions with SH2 and SH3 domains and by means of the adapter proteins Shc and Grb-2; these proteins include mSOS, an activator of the small G-protein Ras, and phospholipase C (*PLC*)γ. The latter enzyme catalyzes the release of the second messenger diacylglycerol (*DAG*; and inositol-1,4,5-trisphosphate, not shown). DAG is also generated along the 7 TMD-R/G protein pathway (*right branch*). DAG stimulates several enzymes of the protein kinase C family (*PKC*). Both Ras and PKC are activators of a cascade of three interconnected protein kinases, i.e. Raf-1, MAPkinase kinase (*MAPKK, MEK*), and the MAPkinase (*MAPK*) isoenzyme Erk. The latter catalyzes the phosphorylation of various target proteins, including transcription factors and enzymes, thereby modulating their activities. This biochemical device of signal processing is a major target of both genotoxic and non-genotoxic carcinogens. As an example, the oncogenic mutation of Ras by the initiating carcinogen DMBA and the short-cut activation of PKC by the tumor promoter TPA, as occurs in experimental skin carcinogenesis are shown. Among the genes activated along these signaling cascades, those for TGFα and cyclooxygenase-2 (COX-2), and among the enzymes phospholipase A_2, the key enzyme of arachidonic acid metabolism, each seem to play a critical part in tumor development. By interacting with the EGF receptor, TGFα activates the left branch of the cascade via a positive feedback loop, whereas arachidonic acid metabolites have been shown to act along the right branch

tumor promotion, initiated cells will, therefore, proliferate faster than the surrounding normal cells and finally gain autonomy. TGFα is indeed frequently elevated in tumor cells (Berkewitz et al. 1996), and an intradermal injection of TGFα has been found to provide a tumor-promoting stimulus in mouse skin (Fürstenberger et al. 1989a). Moreover, targeted overexpression of TGFα in mouse epidermis evokes a hyperplastic response and spontaneous papilloma growth (Dominey et al. 1993) and bypasses the need for *H-ras* mutations (Vassar et al. 1992).

The Eicosanoid Cascade: a Ubiquitous and Versatile Signaling Device

A metabolic process regulated by the MAPkinase cascades at both the transcriptional and the enzymatic level and playing a critical role in mitogenesis, apotosis, and tumor development is the biosynthesis of eicosanoids. Eicosanoids are derivatives of arachidonic acid, which in unstimulated cells is found to be sequestered in phospholipids, from where it is released upon stimulation, for example by wounding or treatment with phorbol esters, or growth factors such as TGFα (Kast et al. 1991, 1993). This means that the eicosanoids are produced only on demand. Thus, the availability of these highly active mediators is directly controlled by the cellular concentrations and activities of the enzymes involved in their biosynthesis. These enzymes can be classified into four major groups: phospholipases for the signal-controlled release of arachidonic acid from membrane phospholipids; prostaglandin-H synthases or cyclooxygenases (COX) for the metabolism of arachidonic acid to prostanoids, i.e., prostaglandins, prostacyclins, and thromboxanes; lipoxygenases (LOX) for the formation of hydroxy-eicosatetraenoic acids (HETEs), leukotrienes, etc.; and cytochromes P450-controlled dioxygenases for epoxidation of arachidonic acid and subsequent reactions (Fig. 3).

Eicosanoids are extremely versatile signal molecules, acting as both inter- and intracellular messengers. Thus, various membrane receptors for prostaglandins, thromboxanes, and leukotrienes have been cloned, which regulate via G-protein interactions the release of second messengers such as cyclic AMP and Ca^{2+} (Narumiya 1996). As intracellular messengers, eicosanoids have been shown to be components of signaling cascades controlling the dynamics of the actin cytoskeleton (Pepellenbosch et al. 1995), and also to bind to and to activate transcription factors (Yu et al. 1995; Forman et al. 1995; Kliewer et al. 1995, 1997; Devchand et al. 1996), in particular those of the PPAR family (peroxisome proliferator-activated receptors).

Eicosanoid biosynthesis is induced along signaling cascades such as the MAP kinase cascades, since activation by the MAP kinase isoenzymes of cytoplasmic phospholipase A_2 provides a major pathway of arachidonic acid release (Lin et al. 1993; Waterman et al. 1996). Thus, the wide variety of extracellular factors acting via such cascades also triggers eicosanoid formation. Moreover, genes coding for enzymes of eicosanoid biosynthesis, such as

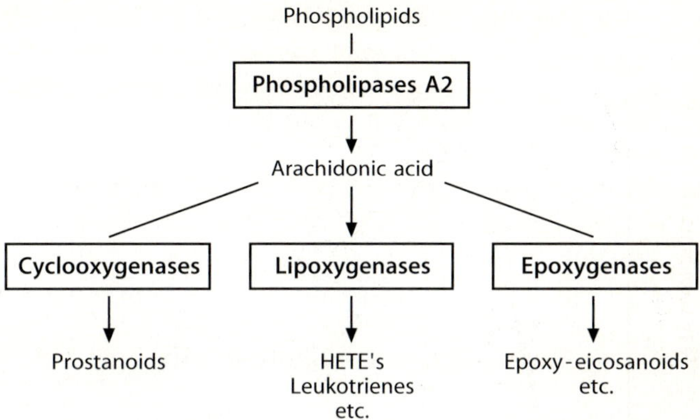

Fig. 3. Major pathways of arachidonic acid metabolism

Table 1. Tissue levels of eicosanoids in the course of multistage carcinogenesis in NMRI mouse skin. Tumors were generated according to the initiation-promotion protocol with 7,12-dimethyl-benz[a]anthracene (DMBA) as initiator and phorbol ester TPA as promoter. The prostaglandin levels were determined by enzyme immunoassay and are given in ng/mg protein. The HETE levels were assayed by GC/MS and are given in ng/g tissue; $N \geq 4$, $SD \leq 25\%$ (Müller-Decker et al. 1995; Krieg et al. 1995). (From Marks et al. 1995)

	Untreated epidermis	Acute hyperplasia[a]	Chronic hyperplasia[b]	Papilloma	Carcinoma
PGE_2	35	85	40	720	800
$PGF_{2\alpha}$	0.5	4	2	15	18
5-HETE	21	36	29	19	1
8-HETE	71	205	789	2764	66
12-HETE	43	57	209	3963	628
15-HETE	74	172	158	322	41

[a] Assayed 6 h (prostaglandins) or 24 h (HETEs) after a single topical application of 10 nmol TPA.
[b] Assayed 2 weeks after 36 applications of 10 nmol TPA, at 3 day intervals.

COX-2, seem to be unter the control of AP-1 transcription factors (Hershman 1996), which are targets of the MAP kinase cascades (see above). Any deregulation of the cascade occuring in the course of tumor formation is therefore expected to result in a pathologic overproduction of prostaglandins, HETEs and other arachidonic acid metabolites. Table 1 shows such a situation for the different stages of tumor development in mouse skin. Considering the biological activities of eicosanoids, an accumulation of such factors in cells may have serious consequences. Thus, prostaglandins have been shown to act both as co-mitogens (Fürstenberger and Marks 1983; Qiao et al. 1995) and as inhibitors of apoptosis (Saiagh et al. 1994; Goetz et al. 1995; Pica et al. 1996; Walker et al. 1997) and may, therefore, stimulate tumor promotion directly. An anti-apoptotic effect has also been described for 12(S)-HETE (Tang et al. 1996), which may also be involved in cancer metastasis (Gao and Honn 1995). 13-Hydroxy-octadecadienoic acid (13-HODE) derived from lino-

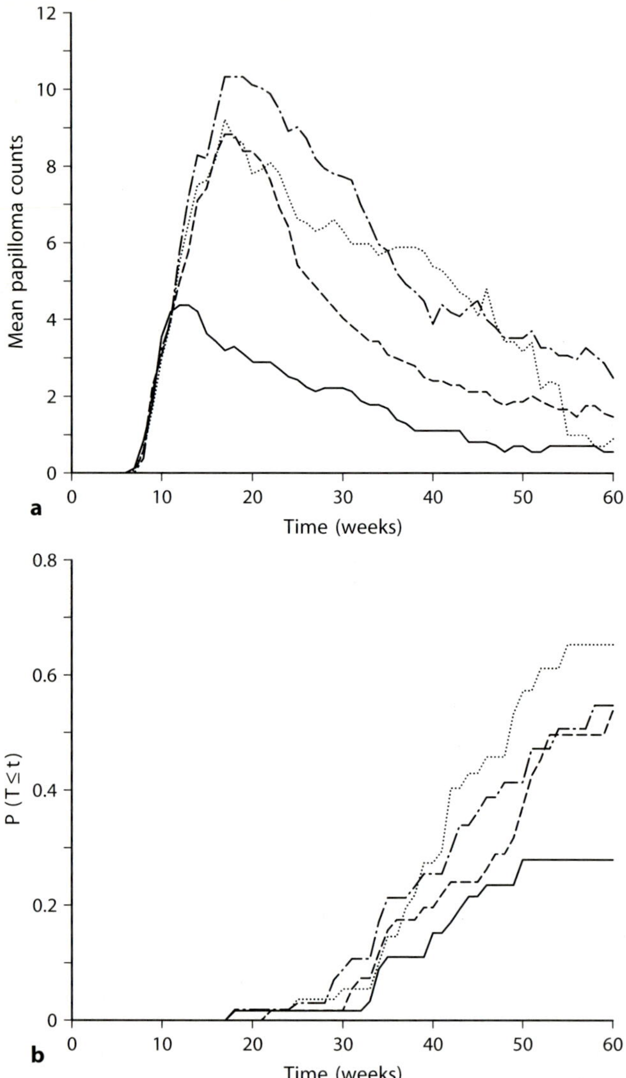

Fig. 4 a, b. Tumor promotion and malignant progression in mouse skin. Tumorigenesis was initiated by a single local application of dimethylbenz[*a*]anthracene at time zero and promoted by local applications of phorbol ester TPA (twice weekly) over a period of 10 (——), 20 (– – –), 30 (······), or 40 (–·–·–) weeks. **a** Development of premalignant lesions (mean papilloma counts per animal); **b** Probability of malignant progression as estimated from the data (Kaplan-Meier estimator of carcinoma occurrence). It is seen that the majority of papillomas exhibit a nonautonomous growth pattern even during prolonged promoter treatment, and that malignant progression occurs regularly and spontaneously even upon cessation of promoter treatment. In the experiment shown, 50% of the autonomous and 4% of all papillomas progressed to carcinomas. From Fürstenberger and Kopp-Schneider (1995)

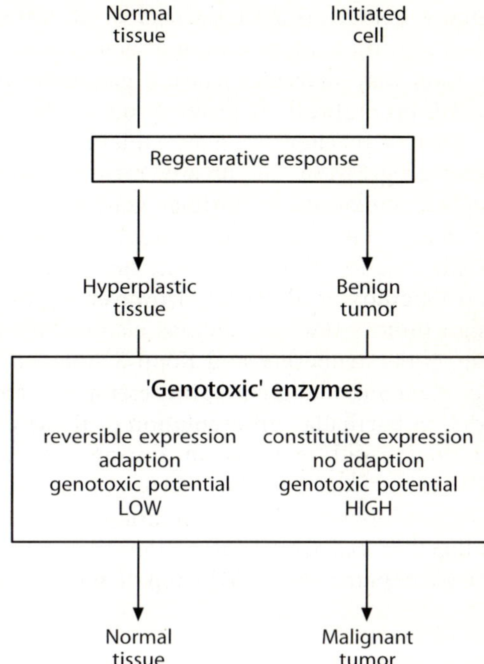

Fig. 5. Malignant progression caused by endogenous factors. It is postulated that while repeated induction of a regenerative response transforms normal tissue into a hyperplastic, the development of benign tumors from initiated cells is promoted. In the course of this process 'genotoxic' enzymes are induced, which catalyze the formation of genotoxic metabolites and by-products. While this induction is reversible in normal cells, which, in addition, may adapt to the stimulus, a constitutive overexpression of such enzymes takes place in tumor cells. This results in a high genotoxic potential, which is thought to facilitate the subsequent mutagenic events required for malignant progression. This concept also explains why chronic induction of tissue regeneration does not have a pronounced tumorigenic effect in normal tissue, i.e. in the absence of initiation (data from Petrusevska et al. 1988). Prime candidates for the status of genotoxic enzymes are cyclooxygenases and the enzymes of lipid peroxidation, such as the arachidonate lipoxygenases. From Marks et al. (1997)

leic acid, another lipoxygenase substrate, enhances signal transduction along the Ras/Raf/Erk cascade in that it attenuates the dephosphorylation of the EGF(TGFa)-receptor (Glasgow et al. 1997). Moreover, the cyclooxygenase- and lipoxygenase-catalyzed metabolic pathways are sources of potentially genotoxic intermediates and by-products, such as free organic radicals, peroxides, reactive oxygen species, and malondialdehyde (Marnett 1994). Reactive oxygen species, in particular, have become prime suspects as endogenous carcinogens (Ames et al. 1995; Wiseman and Halliwell 1996), and cyclooxygenases have even been shown to catalyze the metabolic activation of environmental carcinogens (Marnett 1992).

In addition, 12- and 8-HETE and the corresponding hydroperoxy precursors have been found to induce chromosomal damage in skin cells and probably to mediate the clastogenic effects of phorbol ester tumor promoters in mouse epidermis (Petrusevska et al. 1988; Marks and Fürstenberger 1995). Overactivation of arachidonic acid metabolism in the course of tumor promotion may therefore cause a genotoxic potential to develop in tumor cells, which promotes their progression to malignancy.

Such a mechanism may explain the phenomenon of spontaneous malignant progression. As already mentioned, malignant progression depends on an accumulation of various genetic alterations in initiated cells and can, therefore, be promoted by treatment with genotoxic carcinogens. This also holds true for multistage skin carcinogenesis in mice (Portella et al. 1994; Linardopoulos et al. 1995). However, in this animal model conversion of benign tumors into carcinomas also occurs without any further treatment (see Fig. 4; Fürstenberger and Kopp-Schneider 1995). We have proposed that such spontaneous malignant progression is caused by endogenous genotoxic factors, in particular up-regulation of those produced along the pathways of arachidonic acid metabolism during tumor promotion (Marks et al. 1998). Therefore, the enzymes involved, i.e. lipoxygenases and cyclooxygenases, may be looked upon as potentially 'genotoxic enzymes' (Fig. 5). Another not altogether exclusive explanation of spontaneous malignant progression would be an impairment of DNA repair mechanisms.

Arachidonic Acid Metabolism Provides a Target for Cancer Chemoprevention

The role of signal-regulated mitogenic and apoptotic processes in tumor development gave rise to the concept of cancer chemoprevention and therapy by inhibitors of intracellular signal transduction (Levitzki 1994, 1996; Powis 1994). However, although exciting effects have been observed in experimental systems, it remains open whether or not such drugs can be used in humans, especially for cancer chemoprevention (Gibbs and Oliff 1994). This holds true, in particular, for inhibitors of protein kinases, such as tyrosine kinases and protein kinase C, despite the fact that detailed strategies have been developed for the medical use of such agents (see, e.g. Weinstein 1988; O'Brian et al. 1992; Fry 1994; Grant and Harvis 1996; Basu 1993; Levitzki 1992, 1994, 1996). We were, for instance, unable to prevent phorbol ester-induced tumor promotion in mouse skin by highly specific PKC inhibitors (Gschwendt et al. 1995), and less specific inhibitors, such as staurosporine, even turned out to exhibit some skin tumor-promoting efficacy by themselves (Yoshizawa et al. 1990).

The interruption of tumor development by inhibition of metabolic enzymes that are controlled by signaling cascades has been proved to be more successful. Such enzymes include ornithine decarboxylase and cyclooxygenase.

Expression of ornithine decarboxylase (ODC) is an abundant response to tissue irritation as induced, for instance, by wounding or treatment with phorbol ester tumor promoters (Verma et al. 1988). ODC inhibitors such as

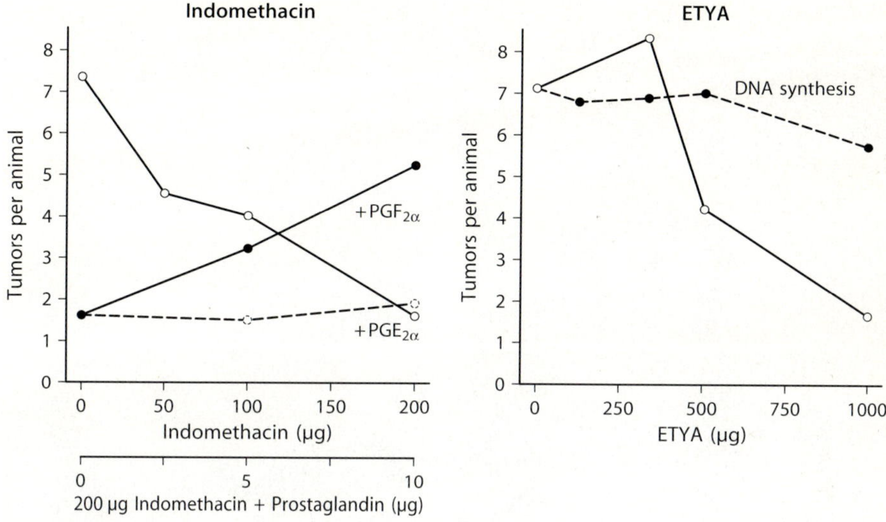

Fig. 6. Inhibition of skin tumor promotion by inhibitors of eicosanoid biosynthesis. Tumor development in NMRI mouse skin was induced according to the initiation-promotion protocol with DMBA as the initiating agent and phorbol ester TPA as the promoting agent. The *left diagram* illustrates the antipromoting effect of topically applied indomethacin (in the doses shown) 30 min before each TPA treatment (*solid line, open circles*). The inhibition caused by 200 µg indomethacin was reversed by simultaneous treatment with prostaglandin $F_{2\alpha}$ (in the doses shown on the *lower abscissa, solid line, black dots*), but not by prostaglandin E_2 (*dotted line;* data from Fürstenberger et al. 1989 b). The *right diagram* shows a similar experiment with ETYA (eicosatetraynoic acid). It can be seen that in the doses applied ETYA inhibited tumor promotion rather than epidermal DNA synthesis (given in arbitrary units). Since the latter is critically dependent on endogenous prostaglandin synthesis (Fürstenberger et al. 1989 b), this result indicates that in these conditions ETYA inhibits lipoxygenase rather than cyclooxygenase activity

difluoromethyl-ornithine (DFMO) are strong inhibitors of tumor development in experimental animals (Verma 1990) and are the subjects of clinical trials (see, e.g., Pegg et al. 1995).

The most promising chemopreventive effects that have been found are those of cyclooxygenase inhibitors. Many of these inhibitors have the great advantage of being immediately available for clinical studies, since they have been in use for many decades as nonsteroidal anti-inflammatory drugs (NSAIDs) against pain, fever, arthritis, and atherosclerotic diseases. The most versatile drug of this group is Aspirin.

Numerous epidemiological and clinical studies have shown that a regular intake of Aspirin or related NSAIDs lowers the general risk of getting colorectal cancer for up to 50% and leads to regression of colon polyps in patients suffering from familial adenomatous polyposis (for reviews see Marnett 1992, 1995; Marcus 1995; Levy 1997; Krishnan and Brenner 1997). These observations are consistent with a large number of animal experiments showing dramatic inhibitory effects of NSAIDs and other inhibitors of arachidonic acid metabolism on tumor development in various organs (Marnett 1992).

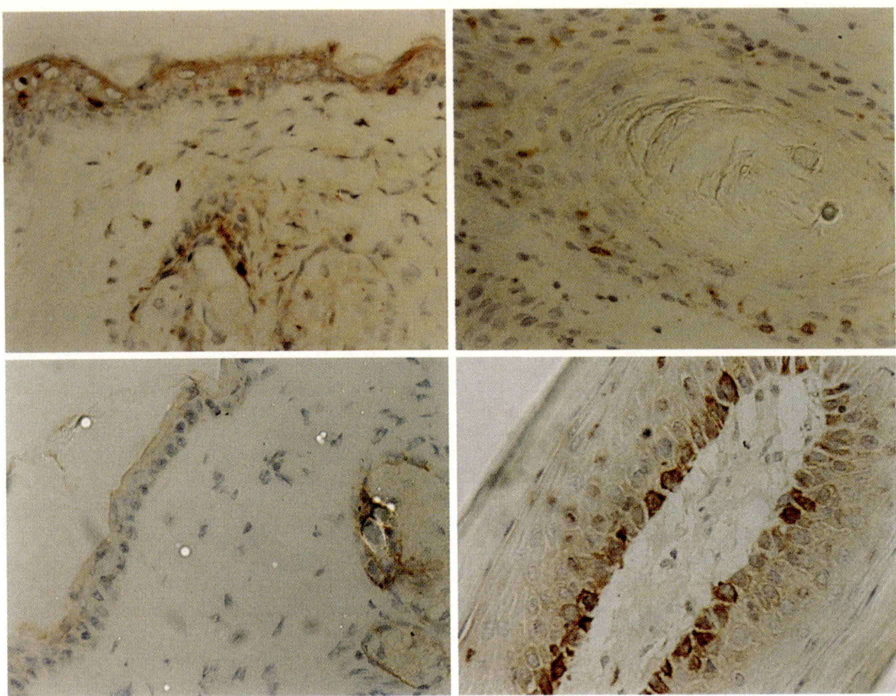

Fig. 7. Expression of cyclooxygenase (COX) isoenzymes in normal mouse skin and premalignant neoplastic lesions. Results of an immunohistochemical analysis of COX-1 (*upper panels*) and COX-2 expression (*lower panels*) in normal epidermis (*left*) and in papillomas generated as described in the legend to Fig. 4 (*right*). COX-positive cells are recognizable by their brown color

Figure 6 showns, as an example, the inhibition of tumor promotion in mouse skin by the NSAID indomethacin. It can be seen that the inhibitory effect could be specifically overcome by low doses of prostaglandin $F_{2\alpha}$, which is overproduced during tumor development (see Table 1). This result proves that in mouse skin the antineoplastic effect of indomethacin is due to an inhibition of prostaglandin biosynthesis (Fürstenberger et al. 1989b). It should be mentioned, however, that for other tissues, including human colon, the situation appears to be less clear, in that cellular mechanisms other than prostaglandin synthesis have been proposed to be the targets of the antineoplastic effects of NSAIDs (Kopp and Gosh 1994; Hanif et al. 1996; Dong et al. 1999; Schwenger et al. 1997).

On the other hand, cancer development both in human colon (Eberhardt et al. 1994; Kargman et al. 1995; Sano et al. 1995; Kutchera et al. 1996) and in experimental animals (Müller-Decker et al. 1995; Williams et al. 1996; Du-Bois et al. 1996) has repeatedly been found to correlate with a constitutive overexpression of COX-2 in tumor cells. In contrast to its isoenzyme, COX-1 (which is a typical 'housekeeping enzyme'), COX-2 is only transiently expressed in most tissues, in particular upon wounding, irritation, hormonal

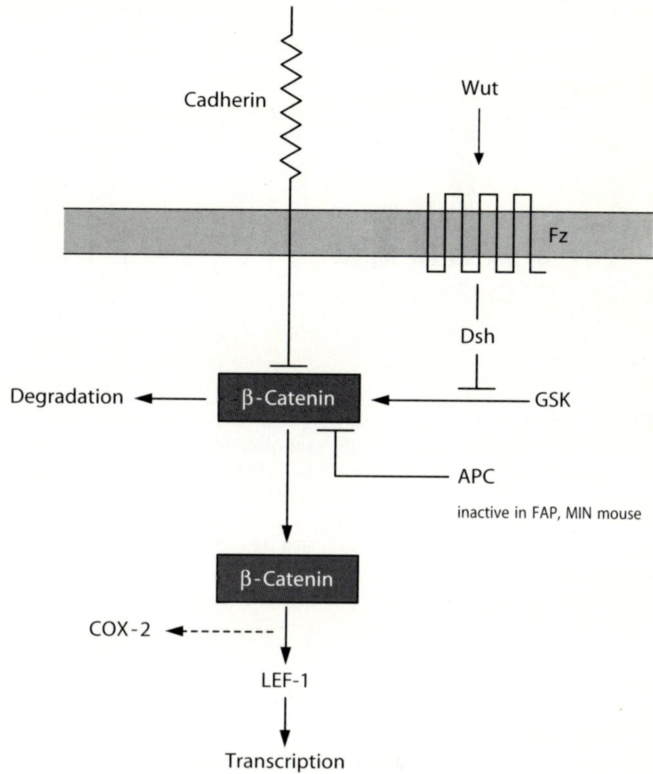

Fig. 8. The β-catenin/Armadillo pathway of signal transduction. It is thought that the protein β-catenin (or Armadillo of *Drosophila*) together with the lef-1 transcription factor controls the expression of several genes. β-Catenin is sequestered in an inactive from by an interaction with cell adhesion molecules of the cadherin family and complex formation with the so-called APC (adenomatous polyposis coli) suppressor protein. Moreover, in these conditions degradation of β-catenin is promoted by glycogen synthase kinase (GSK)-catalyzed phosphorylation. Stabilization and activation of β-catenin seems to occur by inhibition of GSK induced by growth factors of the Wnt family via the transmembrane receptor Fz ('frizzled') and the protein Dsh ('dishevelled'). The *APC* gene is deleted in polyposis patients (FAP, familial adenomatous polyposis) and MIN mice, resulting in spontaneous intestinal tumorigenesis. A major event in APC-deficient cells is an overexpression of COX-2, which is causally related to tumor development. The mechanism of COX-2 expression via the β-catenin/Armadillo pathway is not known

stimulation, and treatment with tumor promoters, for example (Hershman 1996). This is also true for mouse epidermis, where COX-2 expression is transiently induced upon a single treatment with the tumor promoter TPA and becomes constitutive in papillomas and carcinomas (Müller-Decker et al. 1995). While COX-1 expression is scattered throughout the epithelium in both normal and neoplastic epidermis, COX-2 overexpression is restricted to the proliferative cell compartment of papilloma epidermis (Fig. 7).

The constitutive overexpression of COX-2 in tumors represents a pathologic situation, for which different explanations can be proposed. In mouse skin papillomas generated according to the initiation-promotion protocol,

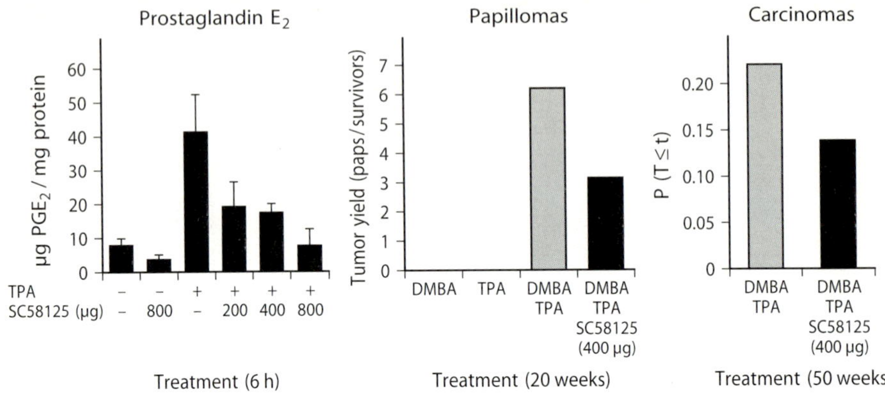

Fig. 9. Suppression of prostaglandin formation and tumor development by a specific COX-2 inhibitor in mouse skin. Tumor development in the skin of mice (strain NMRI) was initiated and promoted as described in the legend to Fig. 4. The COX-2 inhibitor SC58125 (Searle-Monsanto, St. Louis, Mo.) was topically applied in acetone solution 30 min before each TPA application. The diagrams show the effects of different treatments on the epidermal prostaglandin E₂ level (*left diagram*) as determined 6 h after a single TPA application, i.e. at the time of maximal COX-2 induction (Müller-Decker et al. 1995) and on the development of epidermal papillomas (*middle diagram*) and carcinomas (*right diagram*). Each treatment was administered to 80 animals. The carcinoma incidence is expressed as in Fig. 4. (See also Fürstenberger and Kopp-Schneider 1995)

TGFα permanently produced along a deregulated Ras/Raf/Erk cascade probably induces COX-2 expression via an autocrine mechanism leading to a permanent activation of the *COX-2* gene (see Fig. 2; Hershman 1996; Kutchera et al. 1996).

In human colon polyps a direct relationship between COX-2 expression and the *APC* gene seems to exist. *APC* (adenomatous polyposis coli) is a suppressor gene found to be inactivated in polyposis patients at an early stage of tumor development (Kinzler and Vogelstein 1996). In colon cells the APC protein negatively regulates the so-called *β*-catenin/Armadillo signaling cascade which – at least in *Drosophila* and *Xenopus* – is controlled by growth factors of the Wnt family (Fig. 8) and differs completely from other signaling cascades, such as the MAP kinase cascades (Gumbiner 1995, 1997). Gene knockout experiments with MIN mice (MIN = multiple intestinal neoplasia), which are hereditarily defective in *APC* (Dove et al. 1995), have provided strong evidence that in intestinal cells COX-2 expression is somehow controlled along the *β*-catenin/Armadillo pathway, and that a causal relationship exists between *APC* inactivation, tumor development and COX-2 overexpression (Oshima et al. 1996). Thus, in intestinal cells the deletion of a suppressor gene seems to result in a 'self-promotion' of tumor development (Prescott and White 1996). The relationship between *APC* and COX-2 expression in other organs, in particular in mouse skin undergoing multistage carcinogenesis, has not yet been investigated.

The concept of an involvement of COX-2 in tumorigenesis is strongly supported by inhibitor experiments. While the customary NSAIDs inhibit both

COX isoenzymes, highly selective COX-2 inhibitors have recently been developed. Such inhibitors partially suppress intestinal tumorigenesis in rats (Reddy et al. 1996) and MIN mice (Oshima et al. 1996) and skin tumorigenesis in NMRI mice (Fig. 9), and they inhibit the proliferation of human colon carcinoma cells transplanted onto nude mice (Sheng et al. 1997). Conversely, overexpression of COX-2 in such cells results in an increased metastatic potential (Tsujii et al. 1997). Moreover, COX-2-overexpressing rat colon cells are less sensitive to apoptosis-inducing agents (Tsujii and DuBois 1995). It remains to be shown whether the well-known antineoplastic effect of retinoids is also due to a suppression of COX-2 activity, in this case at the transcriptional level, as recently proposed on the basis of cell culture studies (Mestre et al. 1997).

Open Questions and Future Perspectives

Both animal experiments and clinical data clearly show that NSAID treatment interrupts tumor development at a rather early stage but becomes ineffective at later stages, in particular at the malignant stage. Moreover, withdrawal of the drug results in a regrowth of tumors, indicating that neoplastic 'stem cells' carrying oncogenic mutations have not been eradicated. This is exactly the effect to be expected from an agent that inhibits tumor promotion. For successful cancer chemoprevention NSAID treatment must therefore be started at an age when the cancer risk is beginning to rise, and probably continued for the rest of the person's life. Such a situation makes strict control of side effects mandatory, which for many NSAIDs is expected to prove quite practicable.

COX-2 inhibitors are expected to be especially suitable for cancer chemoprevention, since they lack the side effects of the customary NSAIDs (Masferrer et al. 1994). On the other hand, gene knockout experiments have provided evidence that COX-1 is also involved in tumor development, at least as far as the mouse skin model is concerned (Tiano et al. 1997).

Notwithstanding this and several other unanswered questions, in particular about the optimal dose and time-schedule of administration, NSAID treatment certainly provides a most attractive and promising measure of cancer chemoprevention. A major question is whether for man this method is restricted to tumors of the digestive tract or may have a broader applicability, as indicated by preliminary epidemiological data and by animal experiments. The latter possibility would imply that a deregulation of arachidonic acid metabolism is a more general cause of tumor promotion. Moreover, the antineoplastic effect of NSAID treatment in organs other than the colon may depend critically on the type of the drug and how it is applied. This is shown by the following example.

In collaboration with the Dermatological Clinic of the University of Rostock, we have started a study on the role of arachidonic acid metabolism in

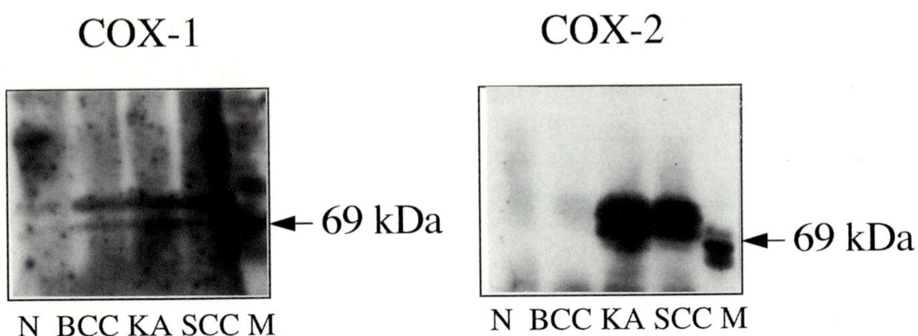

Fig. 10. Cyclooxygenase isoenzyme expression in normal and neoplastic human epidermis. Result of an immunoblot analysis of COX protein levels in normal epidermis (*N*), a basal cell carcinoma (*BCC*), a keratoacanthoma (*KA*), and a squamous cell carcinoma (*SCC*). Both COX-1 and COX-2 appear as *double bands*. A microsomal preparation from the murine keratinocyte line PDV containing both COX-1 and COX-2 severed as a positive control (*M*; note that the molecular weights of mouse COX are somewhat lower than those of human COX). The apparent increase in COX-1 expression in neoplastic epidermis is not significant. (See Müller-Decker et al. (1995))

human skin carcinogenesis. Preliminary results show an accumulation of prostaglandins and an up-regulation of COX-2 expression, in particular in premalignant lesions, such as actinic keratoses, but also in epidermal tumors (Fig. 10). An upregulation of COX-2 expression in UV-irradiated human skin and a constitutive COX-2 overexpression in human squamous cell carcinomas was recently reported by another group (Pentland et al. 1997). In animal experiments we found Aspirin, even in high doses, was unable to inhibit skin tumor formation when given with the drinking water during the promotion phase. However, topical application of a skin-permeable salicyclic acid derivative exerted a strong antineoplastic effect comparable to that of indomethacin (Fig. 11). These results indicate that human skin cancer is a potential target of chemoprevention by NSAID and that the drug should probably be applied topically rather than by the systemic route. Since the majority of skin tumors develop at light-exposed body sites, topical NSAID treatment might be a feasible measure, in particular for such high-risk groups as outdoor workers and chronically immunosuppressed patients. The latter group has been found to be particularly at risk for rapid and multiple tumor development in the skin and other organs (see, e.g., Goya et al. 1995; Glover et al. 1997).

Another target of chemoprevention by NSAIDs might be lung cancer. There is some, albeit still insufficient, epidemiological evidence for a preventive effect of Aspirin intake in humans (Schreinemachers and Everson 1994). Recently, feeding of the NSAID sulindac has been shown to inhibit lung cancer development in mice treated with 4-(methylnitrosamino)-1-(3-pyridyl)-*1*-butanone (NNK), a constituent of tobacco smoke (Castonguay and Rioux 1997). Whether or not arachidonic acid metabolism is constitutively up-regulated in lung tumor cells has not yet been investigated.

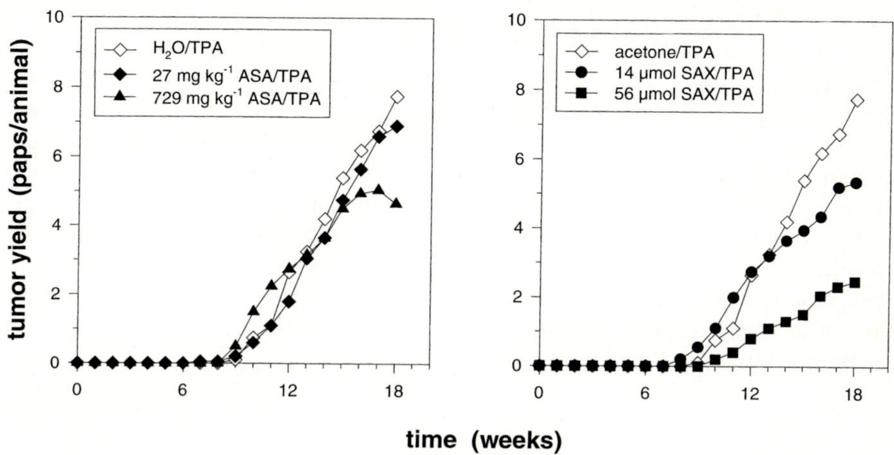

Fig. 11. Effects of systemic application of acetylsalicylic acid (*ASA,* Aspirin) and of the local application of a skin-permeable salicyclic acid derivative, 'SAX,' on experimental skin carcinogenesis. Tumor development was initiated and promoted in the skin of mice (strain NMRI, 80 animals per treatment) as described in the legend to Fig. 4. As shown in the *left diagram* Aspirin (ASA) given with the drinking water over the whole period of the experiment did not inhibit epidermal tumor formation, whereas a skin-permeable salicyclic acid derivative ('SAX') topically applied in acetone solution 30 min before each TPA treatment exhibited a pronounced and dose-dependent antineoplastic effect (*right diagram*). In control experiments it was shown that SAX inhibited prostaglandin synthesis in a cell-free system as effectively as aspirin. This study was performed in collaboration with Bayer AG, Leverkusen, Germany

Among the enzymes for arachidonic acid metabolism, not only cyclooxygenases but also lipoxygenases and phospholipases may provide targets of cancer chemoprevention. Lipoxygenase activity, in particular of the platelet-type 12-LOX (and – in skin – a still ill-defined 8-LOX) becomes up-regulated during tumor development (Krieg et al. 1995), and the corresponding metabolites, i.e., hydroperoxy- and hydroxy-eicosatetraenoic acid, have been shown to induce chromosomal damage (Petrusevska et al. 1988), to inhibit apoptosis (Tang et al. 1996) and to be involved in cancer metastasis (Gao and Honn 1995). Moreover, the lipoxygenase pathways are sources of genotoxic by-products, as already mentioned. In mouse skin, eicosatetraynoic acid (ETYA), a COX and LOX inhibitor, suppresses tumor development and TPA-induced chromosomal damage when topically applied in a low dose that inhibits only LOX (see Fig. 6, Petrusevska et al. 1988), whereas a specific inhibitor of leukotriene biosynthesis has no effect (Fürstenberger et al. 1994). The well-known antineoplastic effects of antioxidants (Slaga 1995) may also be explained, at least partially, by an inhibition of lipoxygenases (Nakadate 1984). These observations urgently call for a more in-depth investigation of the LOX-catalyzed fatty acid metabolism in normal cells and in the course of tumor development, aiming at a possible chemoprevention of human cancer by LOX inhibitors.

Even less is known about a possible role of A_2-type phospholipases (PLA_2) in tumor development, although these enzymes, in particular the highly specific cytoplasmic phospholipases A_2 (cPLA$_2$), catalyze the rate-limiting step of eicosanoid biosynthesis, i.e., the release of free arachidonic acid from phospholipids. Rather unspecific phospholipase inhibitors, such as dibromoacetophenone, have been found to inhibit tumor promotion strongly in mouse skin (Nakadate et al. 1982; Fischer et al. 1982). Moreover, a striking change in cPLA$_2$-catalyzed arachidonic acid metabolism occurs during mouse skin tumor development, in that a phosphatidylcholine-specific enzyme activity is replaced by a phosphatidyl-ethanolamine-specific activity (Marks et al. 1997). The significance of this response is still obscure. In general, much more research is required to elucidate the function of phospholipases in tumorigenesis and the possible role of these enzymes as targets of chemopreventive measures.

Conclusions

Arachidonic acid metabolism is a source of a wide variety of biologically highly active compounds, as well as of genotoxic by-products. An excessive production of such metabolites is a potential hazard, in particular when the protective mechanisms of the cell (such as enzymatic inactivation, provision of anti-oxidants, DNA repair) cannot keep pace with such a deregulation.

A steadily growing body of evidence shows that an overactivation of arachidonic acid metabolism provides a driving force for cancer development, especially for tumor promotion and probably also for malignant progression. In animal experiments inhibitors of arachidonic acid metabolism rank among the most potent antineoplastic agents. The ability of NSAIDs, i.e. inhibitors of prostaglandin synthesis, to interrupt the development of colorectal cancer in humans and other types of neoplasia, in particular skin cancer, efficiently at a premalignant stage in experimental animals is beyond question. Thus, the inhibition of arachidonic acid metabolism seems to be a most promising means of cancer chemoprevention.

Future improvement of this approach depends on the answers to a series of open questions. These include:
The types of neoplasms that can be prevented by these methods.
The optimal dosage and time-schedule of drug application.
The choice of the most appropriate drugs and route of administration, probably depending on the type of neoplasm.
The management of side-effects.
The possible combination of NSAIDs with specific lipoxygenase and phospholipase A_2 inhibitors and with other chemopreventive agents such as anti-oxidants, vitamins, ODC inhibitors etc.

Animal models such as multistage carcinogenesis in mouse skin are especially well suited to an in-depth investigation of the molecular and cellular mechanism underlying the role of arachidonic acid metabolism in tumor development. Studies on such models may yield some guidance that will be useful in the development of novel chemopreventive measures for human application.

References

Ames BN, Gold LS, Willett WC (1995) The causes and prevention of cancer. Proc Natl Acad Sci USA 92:5258–5265

Balmain A, Brown K (1988) Oncogene activation in chemical carcinogenesis. Adv Cancer Res 51:147–182

Basu A (1993) The potential of PKC as a target for anticancer treatment. Pharmacol Ther 59:257–280

Berkowitz EA, Hissong MA, Lee DC (1996) Transcriptional and post-transcriptional induction of the TGFα gene in transformed rat liver epithelial cells. Oncogene 12:1991–2002

Brown K, Kemp C, Burns P, Balmain A (1994) Importance of genetic alterations in tumour development. Arch Toxicol Suppl 16:253–260

Castonguay A, Rioux N (1997) Inhibition of lung tumorigenesis by sulindac: comparison of two experimental protocols. Carcinogenesis 18:491–496

Coffey RJ, Graves-Deal R, Dempsey PJ, Whitehead RH, Pittelkow MR (1992) Differential regulation of transforming growth factor alpha autoinduction in a nontransformed and transformed epithelial cell. Cell Growth Differ 3:347–354

Denhardt DT (1996) Signal-transducing protein phosphorylation cascades mediated by Ras/Rho proteins in the mammalian cell: the potential from multiplex signaling. Biochem J 318:729–747

Devchand PR, Keller H, Peters JM, Vazquez M, Gonzalez FJ, Wahli W (1996) The PPARα-leukotriene B4 pathway to inflammation control. Nature 384:39–43

DiGiovanni J (1992) Multistage carcinogenesis in mouse skin. Pharmacol Ther 54:63–128

Dominey AM, Wang XJ, King LE, Nanney LB, Gagne TA, Sellheyer K, Bundman DS, Longley MA, Rothnagel JA, Greenhalgh DA (1993) Targeted overexpression of transforming growth factor alpha in the epidermis of transgenic mice elicits hyperplasia, hyperkeratosis, and spontaneous papillomas. Cell Growth Differ 4:1071–1082

Dong Z, Huang C, Brown RE, Ma WY (1997) Inhibition of activator protein 1 activity and neoplastic transformation by aspirin. J Biol Chem 272:9962–9970

Dove WF, Gould KA, Luango C, Moser AR, Shoemaker AR (1995) Emergent issues in the genetics of intestinal neoplasia. Cancer Surv 25:335–355

DuBois RN, Radhika A, Reddy BS, Entingh AJ (1996) Increased cyclooxygenase-2 levels in carcinogen-induced rat colonic tumors. Gastroenterology 110:1259–1262

Eberhart CE, Coffey RJ, Radhika A, Giardiello FM, Ferrenbach S, DuBois RN (1994) Up-regulation of cyclooxygenase-2 gene expression in human colorectal adenomas and adenocarcinomas. Gastroenterology 107:1183–1188

Fischer SM, Mills GD, Slaga TJ (1982) Inhibition of mouse skin tumor promotion by several inhibitors of arachidonic acid metabolism. Carcinogenesis 3:1243–1245

Forman BM, Tontonoz P, Chen J, Brun RP, Spiegelman BM, Evans RM (1995) 15-Deoxy-$\Delta^{12,14}$-prostaglandin J$_2$ is a ligand for the adipocyte differentiation factor PPARγ. Cell 83:803–812

Fry DW (1994) Protein tyrosine kinases as therapeutic targets in cancer chemotherapy and recent advances in the development of new inhibitors. Exp Opin Invest Drugs 3:577–595

Fürstenberger G, Marks F (1983) Growth stimulation and tumor promotion in skin. J Invest Dermatol 81:157 s–162 s

Fürstenberger G, Kopp-Schneider A (1995) Malignant progression of papillomas induced by the initiation-promotion protocol in NMRI mouse skin. Carcinogenesis 16:61–69

Fürstenberger G, Czuk-Glänzer BI, Marks F, Keppler D (1994) Phorbol ester-induced leukotriene biosynthesis and tumor promotion in mouse epidermis. Carcinogenesis 15:2823–2827

Fürstenberger G, Rogers M, Schnapke R, Bauer G, Höfler P, Marks F (1989a) Stimulatory role of transforming growth factors in multistage skin carcinogenesis: possible explanation for the tumor-inducing effect of wounding in initiated NMRI mouse skin. Int J Cancer 43:915–921

Fürstenberger G, Gross M, Marks F (1989b) Eicosanoids and multistage carcinogenesis in NMRI mouse skin: role of prostaglandins E and F in conversion (first stage of tumor promotion) and promotion (second stage of tumor promotion). Carcinogenesis 10:91–96

Gao X, Honn KV (1995) Biological properties of 12(S)-HETE in cancer metastasis. Adv Prostaglandin Thromboxane Leukot Res 23:439–444

Gaya SB, Rees AJ, Lechler RI, Williams G, Mason PD (1995) Malignant disease in patients with long-term renal transplants. Transplantation 59:1705–1709

Goetz EJ, An S, Zeng L (1995) Specific suppression by prostaglandin E2 of activation-induced apoptosis of human CD4+CD8+ T lymphoblasts. J Immunol 154:1041–1047

Gibbs JB, Oliff A (1994) Pharmaceutical research in molecular oncology. Cell 79:193–198

Glasgow WC, Hui R, Everhart AL, Jayawickreme, Angerman-Stewart J, Han BB, Eling TE (1997) The linoleic acid metabolite, 13(S)-hydroxyoctadecadienoic acid, augments the epidermal growth factor receptor signaling pathway by attenuation of receptor dephosphorylation. Differential response in Syrian hamster embryo tumor suppressor phenotypes. J Biol Chem 272:19269–19276

Glick AB, Sporn MB, Yuspa SH (1991) Altered regulation of TGF-beta 1 and TGF alpha in primary keratinocytes and papillomas expressing v-Ha-ras. Mol Carcinog 4:210–219

Glover MT, Deeks JJ, Raftery MJ, Cunningham J, Leigh IM (1997) Immunosuppression and risk of non-melanoma skin cancer in renal transplant recipients. Lancet 349:398

Grant S, Jarvis WD (1996) Modulation of drug-induced apoptosis by interruption of the protein kinase C signal transduction pathway: a new therapeutic strategy. Clin Cancer Res 2:1915–1920

Grasso P, Sharratt M, Cohen AJ (1991) Role of persistent, non-genotoxic tissue damage in rodent cancer and relevance to humans. Annu Rev Pharmacol Toxicol 31:253–287

Gschwendt M, Fürstenberger G, Leibersperger H, Kittstein W, Lindner D, Rudolph C, Barth H, Kleinschroth J, Marmé D, Schächtele C, Marks F (1995) Lack of an effect of novel inhibitors with high specificity for protein kinase C on the action of the phorbol ester TPA on mouse skin in vivo. Carcinogenesis 16:107–111

Gumbiner BM (1995) Signal transduction by β-catenin. Curr Opin Cell Biol 7:634–640

Gumbiner BM (1997) A balance between β-catenin and APC. Curr Biol 7:R443–R446

Hanif R, Pittas A, Feng Y, Koutsos MI, Qiao L, Staiano-Coico L, Shiff SI, Rigas B (1996) Effects of nonsteroidal antiinflammatory drugs on proliferation and on induction of apoptosis in colon cancer cells by a prostaglandin-independent pathway. Biochem Pharmacol 52:237–245

Hershman HR (1996) Prostaglandin synthase 2. Biochim Biophys Acta 1299:125–140

Imamoto A, Beltran LM, DiGiovanni J (1991) Evidence for autocrine/paracrine growth stimulation by transforming growth factor-alpha during the process of skin tumor promotion. Mol Carcinog 4:52–60

Kargman S, O'Neill G, Vickers P, Evans J, Mancini J, Jothy S (1995) Expression of prostaglandin G/H synthase-1 and -2 protein in human colon cancer. Cancer Res 55:2556–2559

Karin M, Liu Z, Zandi E (1997) AP-1 function and regulation. Curr Opin Cell Biol 9:240–246

Kast R, Fürstenberger G, Marks F (1991) Activation of a keratinocyte phospholipase A2 by bradykinin and 4β-phorbol 12-myristate 13-acetate. Eur J Biochem 202:941–950

Kast R, Fürstenberger G, Marks F (1993) Activation of a cytosolic phospholipase A2 by transforming growth factor α in HEL-30 keratinocytes. J Biol Chem 268:16795–16802

Kelloff GJ, Boone CW, Crowell JA, Steele VE, Lubet R, Sigman CC (1994) Chemopreventive drug development: Perspectives and progress. Cancer Epidemiol Biomarkers Prev 3:85–98

Kinzler KW, Vogelstein B (1996) Lessons from hereditary colorectal cancer. Cell 87:159–170

Klein SB, Fisher GJ, Jensen TC, Mendelsohn J, Voorhees JJ, Elder JT (1992) Regulation of TGF-alpha expression in human keratinocytes: PKC-dependent and -independent pathways. J Cell Physiol 151:326–336

Kliewer SA, Lenhard JM, Willson TM, Patel I, Morris DC, Lehmann JM (1995) A prostaglandin J_2 metabolite binds peroxisome proliferator-activated receptor γ and promotes adipocyte differentiation. Cell 83:813–819

Kliewer SA, Sundseth SS, Jones SA, Brown PJ, Wisely GB, Koble CS, Devchand P, Wahli W, Willson TM, Lenhard JM, Lehmann JM (1997) Fatty acids and eicosanoids regulate gene expression through direct interactions with peroxisome proliferator-activated receptors α and γ. Proc Natl Acad Sci USA 94:4318–4323

Kopp E, Gosh S (1994) Inhibition of NF-κB sodium salicylate and aspirin. Science 265:956–959

Krieg P, Kinzig A, Ress-Löschke M, Vogel S, Vanlandingham B, Stephan M, Lehmann WD, Marks F, Fürstenberger G (1995) 12-Lipoxygenase isoenzymes in mouse skin tumor development. Mol Carcinog 14:118–129

Krishnan K, Brenner DE (1994) Nonsteroidal anti-inflammatory drugs (NSAIDs) in colorectal cancer chemoprevention. Cancer J 10:10–16

Kutchera W, Jones DA, Matsunami N, Groden J, McIntyre TM, Zimmerman GA, White RL, Prescott SM (1996) Prostaglandin H synthase 2 is expressed abnormally in human colon cancer: evidence for a transcriptional effect. Proc Natl Acad Sci 93:4816–4820

Levitzki A (1992) Tyrphostins: tyrosine kinase blockes as novel antiproliferative agents and dissectors of signal transduction. FASEB J 6:3275–3282

Levitzki A (1994) Signal-transduction therapy. Eur J Biochem 226:1–13

Levitzki A (1996) Targeting signal transduction for disease therapy. Curr Opin Cell Biol 8:239–244

Levy GN (1997) Prostaglandin H synthases, nonsteroidal anti-inflammatory drugs, and colon cancer. FASEB J 11:234–247

Lin LL, Wartmann M, Lin AY, Knopf JL, Seth A, Davis RJ (1993) cPLA2 is phosphorylated and activated by MAPkinase. Cell 72:269–278

Linardopoulos S, Street AJ, Quelle DE, Parry D, Peters G, Sherr CJ, Balmain A (1995) Deletion and altered regulation of p16 (INK4a) and p15 (INK4b) in undifferentiated mouse skin tumors. Cancer Res 55:5168–5172

Marcus AJ (1995) Aspirin as prophylaxis against colorectal cancer. N Engl J Med 333:656–658

Marks F, Fürstenberger G (1995) Tumor promotion in skin. In: Arcos JC (ed) Chemical induction of cancer. Birkhäuser, Boston, pp 125–160

Marks F, Gschwendt M (1995) Protein kinase C and skin tumor promotion. Mutat Res 333:161–172

Marks F, Fürstenberger G, Heinzelmann T, Müller-Decker K (1995) Mechanisms in tumor promotion: guidance for risk assessment and cancer chemoprevention. Toxicol Lett 82/83:907–917

Marks F, Gschwendt M (1996) Protein kinase C. In: Marks F (ed) Protein phosphorylation. VCH, Weinheim, pp 81–116

Marks F, Müller-Decker K, Fürstenberger G (1998) Eicosanoids as endogenous mediators of carcinogenesis and reporters of skin toxicity: cancer chemoprevention by inhibitors of arachidonic acid metabolism. In: Reiss C, Parvez H (eds) Advances in molecular toxicology (1996–97). VSP International Science Press, Zeist

Marnett LJ (1992) Aspirin and the potential role of prostaglandins in colon cancer. Cancer Res 52:5575–5589

Marnett LJ (1994) Generation of mutagens during arachidonic acid metabolism. Cancer Metastasis Rev 13:303–308

Marnett LJ (1995) Aspirin and related nonsteroidal anti-inflammatory drugs as chemopreventive agents against colon cancer. Prev Med 24:103–106

Masferrer JL, Zweifel BS, Manning PT, Hauser SO, Leaky KM, Smith WG, Isakson PC, Seibert K (1994) Selective inhibition of inducible cyclooxygenase 2 in vivo is antiinflammatory and nonulcerogenic. Proc Natl Acad Sci USA 91:3228–3282

Mestre JR, Subbaramaiah K, Sacks PG, Schantz SP, Tanabe T, Inoue H, Dannenberg AJ (1997) Retinoids suppress phorbol ester-mediated induction of cyclooxygenase-2. Cancer Res 57:1081–1085

Müller-Decker K, Scholz K, Marks F, Fürstenberger G (1995) Differential expression of prostaglandin H synthase isozymes during multistage carcinogenesis in mouse epidermis. Mol Carcinog 12:31–41

Nakadate T, Yamamoto S, Iseki H, Sonoda S, Takemura S, Ura A, Hosoda Y, Kato R (1982) Inhibition of TPA-induced tumor promotion by nordihydroguaiaretic acid, a lipoxygenase inhibitor, and p-bromophenacyl bromide, a phospholipase A_2 inhibitor. Gann 73:841–843

Nakadate T, Yamamoto S, Aizu E, Kato R (1984) Effects of flavonoids and antioxidants on 12-O-tetradecanoyl-phorbol-13-acetate-caused epidermal ornithine decarboxylase induction and tumor promotion in relation to lipoxygenase inhibition by these compounds. Gann 75:214–222

Narumiya S (1996) Prostanoid receptors and signal transduction. Prog Brain Res 113:231–241

Naumann U, Hoffmeyer A, Flory E, Rapp UR (1996) Raf protein serine/threonine kinases. In: Marks F (ed) Protein phosphorylation. VCH, Weinheim, pp 203–236

O'Brian CA, Ward NE, Ioannides CG, Dong Z (1992) Potential strategies of chemoprevention through modulation of protein kinase C activity. In: Steele VE, Boone CW, Stoner GD, Kelloff GJ (eds) Cellular and molecular targets for chemoprevention. CRC Press, Bocan Raton, pp 161–172

Oshima M, Dinchuk JE, Kargman SL, Oshima H, Hancock B, Kwong E, Trzaskos JM, Evans JF, Taketo MM (1996) Suppression of intestinal polyposis in APC$^{\Delta716}$ knockout mice by inhibition of cyclooxygenase 2 (COX-2). Cell 87:803–809

Pegg AE, Shantz LM, Coleman CS (1995) Ornithine decarboxylase as a target for chemoprevention. J Cell Biochem Suppl 22:132–138

Pentland AP, Masferrer J, Hale P, Gresham A, Buckman S (1997) Induction of COX-2 by UVB: potential role in the development of human skin cancer. J Invest Dermatol 108:547

Pepellenbosch MP, Qui RG, de Vries-Smits AMM, Tertoolen LGJ, deLaat SW, McCormick F, Hall A, Symons MH, Bos JL (1995) Rac mediates growth factor-induced arachidonic acid release. Cell 81:849–856

Petrusevska RT, Fürstenberger G, Marks F, Fusenig N (1988) Cytogenetic effects caused by phorbol ester tumor promoters in primary mouse keratinocyte cultures: correlation with the convertogenic activity of TPA in multistage skin carcinogenesis. Carcinogenesis 9:1207–1215

Pica F, Franzese O, D'Onofrio C, Bonmassar E, Favalli C, Garaci E (1996) Prostaglandin E_2 induces apoptosis in resting immature and mature human lymphocytes: a c-myc-dependent and Bcl-2 independent associated pathway. J Pharmacol Exp Ther 277:1793–1800

Portella G, Liddell J, Crombie R, Haddow S, Clarke M, Stoler AB, Balmain A (1994) Molecular mechanisms of invasion and metastasis during mouse skin tumor progression. Invasion Metastasis 14:1–6

Powis G (1994) Signaling pathways as targets for anticancer drug development. Pharmacol Ther 62:57–95

Prescott SM, White RL (1996) Self-promotion? Intimate connections between APC and prostaglandin H synthase-2. Cell 87:783–786

Qiao L, Kozoni V, Tsioulias GJ, Koutsos MI, Hanif R, Shiff SJ, Rigas B (1995) Selected eicosanoids increase the proliferation rate of human colon carcinoma cell lines and mouse colonocytes in vivo. Biochim Biophys Acta 14:215–223

Reddy BS, Rao CV, Seibert K (1996) Evaluation of cyclooocygenase-2 inhibitor for potential chemopreventive properties in colon carcinogenesis. Cancer Res 56:4566–4569

Saiagh S, Rigal D, Monier JC (1994) Effects of PGE 2 upon differentiation and programmed cell death of suspension cultured CD 4-CD 8-thymocytes. Int J Immunopharmacol 16:775–786

Sano H, Kawahito Y, Wilder RL, Hashiramoto A, Mukai S, Asai K, Kimura S, Kato H, Kondo M, Hla T (1995) Expression of cyclooxygenase-1 and -2 in human colorectal cancer. Cancer Res 55:3785–3789

Schreinemachers DM, Everson RB (1994) Aspirin use and lung, colon, and breast cancer incidence in a prospective study. Epidemiology 5:138–146

Schwarz M (1995) Tumor promotion in liver. In: Arcos JC (ed) Chemical induction of cancer. Birkhäuser, Boston, pp 161–179

Schwenger P, Bellosta P, Vietor I, Basilico C, Skolnik EY, Vilcek J (1997) Sodium salicylate induces apoptosis via p38 mitogen-activated protein kinase but inhibits tumor necrosis factor-induced c-Jun N-terminal kinase/stress-activated protein kinase activation. Proc Natl Acad Sci USA 94:2869–2873

Seger R, Krebs EG (1995) The MAPK signaling cascade. FASEB J 9:726–735

Shaw IC, Jones HB (1994) Mechanisms of non-genotoxic carcinogenesis. Trends Pharmacol Sci 15:89–93

Sheng H, Shao J, Kirkland SC, Isakson P, Coffey RJ, Morrow J, Beauchamp RD, DuBois RN (1997) Inhibition of human colon cancer cell growth by selective inhibition of cyclooxygenase-2. J Clin Invest 99:2254–2259

Slaga TJ (1995) Inhibition of the induction of cancer by anti-oxidants. Adv Exp Med Biol 369:167–174

Tang DG, Chen JQ, Honn KV (1996) Arachidonate lipoxygenases as essential regulators of cell survival and apoptosis. Proc Natl Acad Sci USA 93:5241–5246

Tiano H, Chulada P, Spalding J, Lee C, Loftin C, Mahler J, Morham S, Langenbach R (1997) Effects of cyclooxygenase deficiency on inflammation and papilloma development in mouse skin. Proc Am Assoc Cancer Res 38:257

Treisman R (1996) Regulation of transcription by MAPkinase cascades. Curr Opin Cell Biol 8:205–215

Tsujii M, DuBois RN (1995) Alterations in cellular adhesion and apoptosis in epithelial cells overexpressing prostaglandin endoperoxide synthase-2. Cell 83:493–501

Tsujii M, Kawano S, DuBois RN (1997) Cyclooxygenase-2 expression in human colon cancer cells increases metastatic potential. Proc Natl Acad Sci USA 94:3336–3340

Vassar R, Hutton ME, Fuchs E (1992) Transgenic overexpression of TGFα bypasses the need for c-Ha-ras mutations in mouse skin tomorigenesis. Mol Cell Biol 12:4643–4653

Verma AK (1990) Inhibition of tumor promotion by DL-alpha-difluoromethylornithine, a specific irreversible inhibitor of ornithine decarboxylase. Basic Life Sci 52:195–204

Verma AK, Hsieh JT, Pong PC (1988) Mechanisms involved in ornithine decarboxylase induction by 12-O-tetradecanoylphorbol-13-acetate, a potent mouse skin tumor promoter and an activator of protein kinase C. Adv Exp Med Biol 250:273–290

Walker BA, Rocchini C, Boone RH, Jacobson MA (1997) Adenosine A2a receptor activation delays apoptosis in human neutrophils. J Immunol 158:2926–2931

Wang HG, Rapp UR, Reed JC (1996) Bcl-2-targets the protein kinase Raf-1 to mitochondria. Cell 87:1–20

Waterman WH, Molski TF, Huang CK, Adams JL, Sha'afi RI (1996) Tumour necrosis factor-alpha-induced phosphorylation and activation of cytosolic phospholipase A2 are abrogated by an inhibitor of the p38 mitogen-activated protein kinase cascade in human neutrophils. Biochem J 319:17–20

Weinstein IB (1988) Strategies for inhibiting multistage carcinogenesis based on signal transduction pathways. Mutat Res 202:413–420

Williams CS, Luongo C, Radhika A, Zhang T, Lamps LW, Nanney LB, Beauchamp RD, DuBois RN (1996) Elevated cyclooxygenase-2 levels in Min mouse adenomas. Gastoenterology 111:1134–1140

Wiseman H, Halliwell B (1996) Damage to DNA by reactive oxygen and nitrogen species: role in inflammatory diseases and progression to cancer. Biochem J 313:17–29

Yoshizawa SH, Fujiki, Sugori H, Suganuma M, Nakayasu M, Matsushima R, Sugimura T (1990) Tumor-promoting activity of staurosporine, a potent protein kinase inhibitor, on mouse skin. Cancer Res 50:4974–4978

Yu K, Bayonna W, Kallen CB, Harding HP, Ravera CP, McMahon G, Brown M, Lazar MA (1995) Differential activation of peroxisome proliferator-activated receptors by eicosanoids. J Biol Chem 270:23975–23983

III. Identification of Meaningful High Risk Groups for Cancer Chemoprevention

Prognostic Implications of Cancer Susceptibility Genes: Any News?

R. J. Scott[1] and H. H. Sobol[2]

[1] Hunter Area Pathology Service, Locked Bag 1, New Lambton,
2310 New South Wales, Australia
[2] Genetic Oncology Department/INSERM CRI 9703,
Institut Jean-Paoli Calmettes, 232, Bd. St. Marguerite, F-13009 Marseille, France

Abstract

Recent advances in our understanding of the genetic basis of several inherited predispositions to cancer have raised the possibility that there may be differences in prognosis between patients harbouring genetic susceptibilities to cancer and persons presenting with sporadic disease. The two best studied models of inherited susceptibilities to cancer will be considered, those of colorectal cancer and familial breast cancer. Familial colorectal cancer can be subdivided into essentially two groups: familial adenomatous polyposis and hereditary non-polyposis colorectal cancer. Familial breast cancer can be subdivided into three groups: those that can be accounted for by mutations in the breast cancer susceptibility gene *BRCA 1*, families harbouring mutations in *BRCA 2* and families where neither *BRCA 1* nor *BRCA 2* appear to be involved. In this chapter several aspects of these inherited cancer predispositions will be discussed and compared with their equivalent sporadic disease counterparts.

Introduction

Inherited susceptibilities to cancer represent model diseases from which inferences can be made concerning the etiology of common malignancies such as breast and colorectal cancer. Several cancer susceptibility genes associated with breast or colorectal cancer development (shown in Table 1) have now been identified, which predispose persons harbouring germline mutations in these genes to a very high probability of developing neoplastic disease at unusually early ages. Cancer susceptibility genes include tumour suppressor genes, oncogenes and genes involved in maintaining genomic integrity. Tumour suppressor genes and genes associated with maintaining genomic integrity will be examined in detail. Oncogenes do not appear to play a major part in inherited predispositions to cancer and appear to be associated more with disease progression than with initiation. The two examples that have

Recent Results in Cancer Research, Vol. 151
Senn/Costa/Jordan (Eds.): Chemoprevention of Cancer
© Springer-Verlag Berlin · Heidelberg 1999

Table 1. Genes associated with breast or colorectal cancer predispositions

Colorectal cancer			
Disease	Gene	Size (bp)	Function
FAP	APC	8972	Beta-catenin regulation
HNPCC	hMSH2	2947	DNA mismatch repair
	hMLH1	2482	DNA mismatch repair
	hPMS1	3063	DNA mismatch repair
	hPMS2	2697	DNA mismatch repair
Peutz-Jeghers	STK11	1301	Serine/threonine kinase
Juvenile polyposis	JP	–	Unknown
Breast cancer			
Disease	Gene	Size (bp)	Function
Breast/ovarian	BRCA1	5711	DNA repair?
Breast/ovarian	BRCA2	10987	DNA repair?
Li-Fraumeni	p53	1179	Cell cycle control
Cowden disease	pten/mmac	1212	Tyrosine kinase
Oestrogen receptor	ER	2092	Receptor
Androgen receptor	AR	3061	Receptor
Ataxia telangiectasia	ATM	9385	PI3 kinase and other functions

been described to date are the proto-oncogenes *RET* and *MET*. The *RET* proto-oncogene has been linked to the development of multiple endocrine neoplasia (Mulligan et al. 1993) and the *MET* oncogene has recently been identified as being integral to the development of inherited clear cell kidney cancer (Schmidt et al. 1997). The recognition that genes existed that acted by suppressing cellular growth has formed the basis of our current concepts of tumour cell development. Tumour suppressor genes have now been identified in many different malignancies and indeed appear to be essential not only for the initiation of disease but also for progression. For quite some time it has been recognised that genes controlling DNA repair are essential for maintaining genomic integrity and hence normal gene expression. Perturbations in DNA repair have been recognised for many years as being associated with an increased likelihood of developing neoplastic disease (Hanawalt 1991). DNA repair errors were considered earlier to be confined to such rare diseases as xeroderma pigmentosum, ataxia telangiectasia and Fanconi anaemia (Robbins et al. 1974; Gatti et al. 1991; Sasaki 1975). These three diseases have been shown to be associated with specific types of DNA repair, including nucleotide excision repair, DNA strand break repair and DNA cross-link repair, respectively. All three of these diseases are rare entities compared with other, more common, malignancies. More recently, a fourth DNA repair group, DNA mismatch repair, has been identified, which is associated with a common cancer predisposition, namely hereditary non-polyposis colorectal cancer (Fischel et al. 1993; Leach et al. 1993).

The identification of different types of genes associated with inherited predispositions to malignancy raises several questions concerning not only the likelihood of disease development, but also whether or not patients inheriting a particular genetic predisposition are likely to behave in a similar way with respect to disease progression, response to treatment and prognosis, to persons who develop disease in the absence of any clear genetic influence. In this chapter three model diseases will be considered, familial adenomatous polyposis, hereditary non-polyposis colorectal cancer, and familial breast cancer.

Familial Adenomatous Polyposis

Familial adenomatous polyposis (FAP) is an autosomal dominantly inherited disease characterized by the appearance of hundreds to thousands of adenomatous polyps that carpet the entire colon and rectum. If left untreated patients are virtually certain to develop colorectal cancer by their 5th decade of life (Bülow 1987). In addition to colorectal adenomas extracolonic disease manifestations present in some patients, which can be benign (such as osteomas, lipomas and hypertrophy of the retinal pigment epithelium), premalignant (adenomas in the upper GI tract) or malignant (desmoid disease).

The identification of of the adenomaotus polyposis coli (*APC*) gene in 1991 (Nishisho et al. 1991; Groden et al. 1991) was a major step forward in our understanding of the development of neoplasia not only in FAP but also in colorectal cancer in general. Along with the identification of the gene it became possible to perform predictive molecular analysis by direct genetic testing (Miyoshi et al. 1992; Fodde et al. 1992). Predictive testing in FAP was a significant advance in the management of patients, as it mean that for the first time a person could be identified accurately before the onset of symptoms. The *APC* gene consists of 15 exons encompassing about 8500 base pairs, exon 15 being one of the largest exons identified to date (about 6500 bp) and encoding a protein of 2843 amino acids (Joslyn et al. 1991). The APC protein homodimerizes and contains a series of heptad repeats, which appear to be essential for the binding to various proteins, such as glycogen synthase kinase (GSK) 3 beta (Rubinfeld et al. 1996), the E1B protein (Su et al. 1995) and *Drosophila* large disks (DLG) protein (Matsumine et al. 1996). Currently it is not known what influence these proteins have on *APC* function or what influence of *APC* has on GSK3beta, E1B or DLG. The precise function of the *APC* gene is not yet fully determined; however, there is sufficient evidence to suggest that *APC* is involved in the regulation of beta catenin (Rubinfeld et al. 1993). Beta catenin, if not tightly controlled, will constitutively stimulate the production of at least two transcription factors (termed Lef 1 and TCF1), which presumably leads to a loss of gene expression control (Korinek et al. 1997).

Since the identification of the *APC* gene phenotype/genotype, correlations between the site of mutation in the *APC* gene and disease types have been forthcoming (see Fig. 1). Mutations occurring at the 5′ end of the gene are associated with a milder phenotype characterized by few colonic polyps and a later age at disease onset than in typical FAP patients (Spirio et al. 1993; Dobbie et al. 1994). Mutations occurring 3′ off codon 157 and before ap-

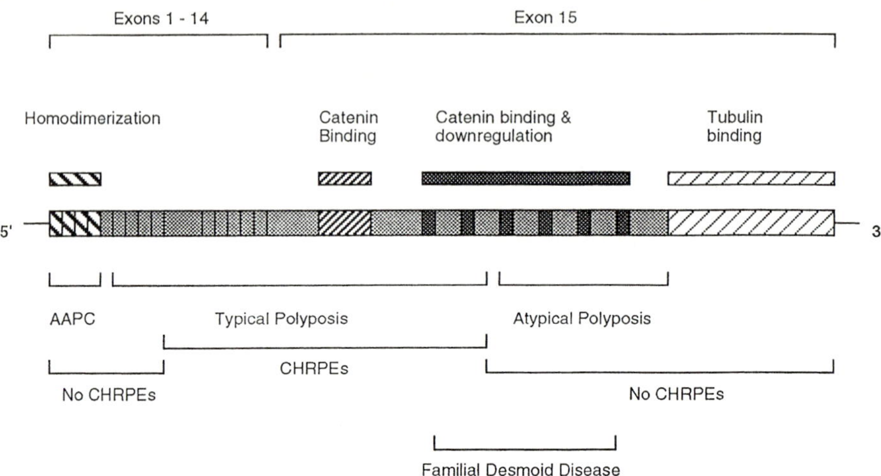

Fig. 1. Schematic representation of the APC gene, indicating the correlation between mutation site (shown under the gene) and expected disease expression, and functional regions of the *APC* gene

proximately codon 1403 (Dobbie et al. 1996) appear to be associated with a more typical FAP phenotype, but one mutation at codon 1309 results in an extremely severe colonic disease phenotype; patients so affected present with thousands of adenomas that completely carpet the colonic mucosa. The risk of developing very early onset colorectal cancer is extremely high, and these patients therefore require regular and frequent screening both before and after colectomy. A prediction of colorectal disease and extracolonic disease can be made with mutations beyond codon 1403, since most families harbouring mutations beyond this site appear to develop other symptoms in addition to colonic disease (Dobbie et al. 1996). Interestingly, mutations that occur towards the 3' end of the gene (that is beyond codon 1597) have similarities with those occurring at the 5' end with respect to colonic disease expression, as they also appear to predispose to a milder phenotype characterized by fewer adenomas, but not necessarily earlier ages of onset (Scott et al. 1995; Friedl et al. 1996; van der Luijt et al. 1996). It remains difficult, however, to determine what percentage of families harbour mutations in the 3' end of the *APC* gene, since in many centres this region is not examined.

Subdivisions with respect to disease can be made when certain particular disease symptoms are considered specifically. Congenital hypertrophy of the retinal pigment epithelium has often been cited as a useful non-invasive marker of carrier status in FAP (Burn et al. 1991). Molecular data indicate that this particular manifestation of FAP is restricted to a region in the *APC* gene that is bounded by exon 9 at the 5' end of the gene and at about the first third of exon 15 in the 3' direction (Caspari et al. 1995; Olschwang et al. 1993). More recently, molecular studies of familial infiltrative fibromatosis (or desmoid disease) have indicated that there is a desmoid cluster region in the *APC* gene; several families have been identified that present with desmoid disease in the presence or absence of colorectal symptoms (Scott et al. 1996; Eccles et al. 1996).

Knowledge of where the genetic defect lies in the *APC* gene can be used to a certain extent as a predictor of disease phenotype. Additional studies using animal models of FAP have revealed that there are modifying genes that also appear to influence disease expression, and it is therefore to be expected that some of these genes will also affect disease expression in man (Dietrich et al. 1994; MacPhee et al. 1995).

Since it has been recognized that FAP is an inherited disorder and that effective clinical management is available to treat colorectal disease, the prognosis of patients harbouring mutations in the *APC* gene has improved significantly. In the absence of any medical intervention life expectancy was in the region of 40 years whereas today, with adequate clinical surveillance and care life expectancy has extended to over 60 years of age (Bülow et al. 1996). The major difficulty facing FAP patients is now no longer the problem of colorectal disease, but the development of extracolonic manifestations, which are usually much more difficult to treat. These include adenomas of the ampulla of Vater, which are surgically challenging and desmoid tumours that tend to be resistant to all forms of treatment. Thus, on the one hand there has been a considerable improvement in the life expectancy of FAP patients, but on the other the prognosis remains poor when additional disease manifestations are considered.

Unfortunately, colorectal cancer remains a problem in FAP for several reasons. Firstly, it is not always possible for patients to be screened regularly, so that their initial presentation is with colorectal cancer. Secondly, approximately 20% of all polyposis coli patients represent new mutations (Miyoshi et al. 1992), implying that a significant number of patients will present without a family history of disease and hence cannot benefit from early screening procedures. It is important, however, that their offspring should be screened, as they will have a high probability of inheriting this new predisposition.

There appears in FAP to be little if any difference in disease progression compared to sporadic colorectal cancer once neoplasia is established suggesting that disease development in sporadic disease is similar to that observed in this inherited syndrome. Two implications can be drawn from this information; one, early screening of affected persons and adequate intervention measures will improve the prognosis of FAP patients and two, early screening protocols for the general population will lead to an overall decrease in colorectal cancer mortality by virtue of the fact that premalignant adenomas can be removed prior to carcinoma development.

The treatment of colonic symptoms of FAP by non-invasive methods has made some progress in recent years. The recognition that the non-steroidal anti-inflammatory drug, Sulindac (otherwise known as Clinoril) is effective in reducing the numbers of adenomas within the colon and rectum may aid in the management of FAP patients (Labayle et al. 1991; Giardiello et al. 1993). Furthermore, it has been suggested by larger studies in sporadic colorectal cancer that low-dose aspirin may also be beneficial in treatment (Giovannucci et al. 1995). An ongoing investigation known as the CAPP (Concerted Action Polyposis Prevention) study organised by Professor John Burn (see end of chapter for address details) is currently assessing the value of an aspirin intervention study for FAP patients, as there are currently no double blind trials determining the efficacy of this agent.

Hereditary Non-Polyposis Colorectal Cancer

Hereditary non-polyposis colorectal cancer (HNPCC) is a synonym for a inherited predisposition encompassing a broader spectrum of neoplastic disease than its name implies. In addition to a familial clustering of colorectal disease, other cancers are frequently observed in HNPCC, including endometrial cancer, upper renal tract cancers and nasopharyngeal cancers (see Table 2 for a complete list). After colorectal cancer, endometrial cancer is the second most common malignancy found in HNPCC families, and together these two diseases account for almost 90% of all cancers (Lynch et al. 1993).

The identification of the genetic basis of this disease has altered the way in which cancer development is perceived. Prior to the identification of DNA mismatch repair genes that are involved in neoplasia it was believed that DNA repair disorders were confined to extremely rare diseases, which were in general inherited in an autosomal recessive manner. Furthermore, alterations in tumour suppressor genes and oncogenes were considered to be essential elements of tumour initiation. DNA mismatch repair genes represented a third category of genes which are integral in tumour formation. This has led to the notion that tumour suppressor genes and oncogenes can be classified as "gatekepper genes", whilst genes associated with genomic integrity are known as "caretaker genes" (Kinzler and Vogelstein 1996). This classification system implies that if a mutation is inherited in a gatekeeper gene, disease will inevitably develop in a given tissue, which is dependent on

Table 2. Cancers frequently observed in hereditary non-polyposis colorectal cancer

Colorectal cancer
Endometrial cancer
Ovarian cancer
Gastric cancer
Cholangiocarcinoma
Upper renal tract cancers
Nasopharyngeal cancer
Glioblastoma multiforme
Hepatobilary tumours
Cancer of the small bowel
Skin cancer
Laryngeal cancer
Breast cancer

the gene in question (a good example being the APC gene in familial adenomatous polyposis). Mutations in caretaker genes change the probability of disease, as these genes are involved in ameliorating the effects of the environment (the genes associated with DNA repair are an example); therefore, pertubations in these genes change the risk of disease development but do not make it a foregone conclusion.

By the end of 1993 two groups had identified a gene that belonged to the DNA mismatch repair complex (Fischel et al. 1993; Leach et al. 1993), and within a few months a second gene has been described (Bronner et al. 1994; Papadopoulos et al. 1994). In total, seven human genes have now been identified (see Table 3), all associated with DNA mismatch repair (MMR), four of which appear to play a central part in disease development, these being hMSH 2, hMLH 1, hPMS 1 and hPMS 2 (Fischel et al. 1993; Kolodner et al. 1995; Papadopoulos et al. 1994, Nicolaides et al. 1994).

The precise mechanism by which the MMR genes achieve their function is not clearly understood and awaits further verification. It is becoming increasingly evident that some of the MMR genes associated with HNPCC, in addition to their MMR function are capable of contributing to other DNA repair processes. The genes hMSH 2 and hPMS 2 have been implicated in a variant of the nucleotide excision repair process, namely, transcription-coupled repair (Mellon et al. 1996); and hMLH 1 has been shown to be involved in meiotic recombination repair (Baker et al. 1996). At a superficial level it appears that mutations in either hMSH 2 or hMLH 1 do not predict any particular phenotype. This is not surprising, as DNA mismatch repair is a cellular housekeeping process such that any perturbation in MMR that leads to a change in repair proficiency would eventuate in a similar phenotype, since it is the functional complex that is ultimately disrupted. There are, however, subtle differences that may be present in families that harbour mutations in hMSH 2 as opposed to those harbouring hMLH 1 changes. In addition, there is evidence to suggest that some types of mutations predispose to a more focused phenotype than others (Rogan et al. 1997). Compared with FAP, HNPCC does not appear to lend itself to genotype/pheno-

Table 3. Conserved mismatch repair genes. Genes indicated in bold face have been shown to be clearly associated with hereditary non-polyposis colorectal cancer

E. coli	S. cerevisiae	H. sapiens
MutS	MSH2	**hMSH2**
	MSH3	hMSH3
	MSH5	MSH5
	MSH6	hMSH6 (GTBP)
MutL	MLH1	**hMLH1**
MutH		
	PMS1	**hPMS2**
	PMS2	**hPMS1**

type correlations, suggesting that other genetic or epigenetic influences may be important in determining a particular phenotype.

There has been an ongoing debate as to whether survival in the case of HNPCC is better than in persons who develop colorectal cancer in the absence of any family history. By evaluating persons known to be harbouring MMR gene mutations it has now become apparent that there is statistically a much better 5-year survival in HNPCC than in sporadic disease, especially when relative gradings are taken into account (Mecklin and Jarvinen 1986). Better survival is not restricted to colonic disease: it is noteworthy that in a series of Turcot cases (brain tumours in association with HNPCC colorectal cancers) survival with glioblastoma multiforme was much better than could be expected from the usual dismal prognosis of this lesion (Hamilton et al. 1995). Caution must be exercised, however, as in a series of Turcot patients reported by Merlo et al. (1996) survival was as expected for this condition.

Since the recognition of MMR as the underlying genetic cause of disease in HNPCC an improvement in morbidity has been reported. In a Finnish series of patients identified as harbouring germline mutations in either hMSH2 or hMLH1, regular colonoscopy and transvaginal ultrasound were used to screen for colorectal and endometrial disease, respectively, which has led to a better survival (Jarvinen et al. 1995). Therefore, it appears that an improvement in morbidity and hence mortality is likely, provided that patients recognize the necessity for regular screening.

Prevention strategies for HNPCC are not as well advanced as those for FAP, but an intervention trial similar to the CAPP study is being conducted with respect to the actions of aspirin in HNPCC patients, the end-point being a reduction in incident cancers over a given time period (contact Professor Burn for details).

Familial Breast Cancer

A family history of breast cancer has been and remains one of the single most important and consistent factors in determining a woman's risk of developing this fatal disease and can to some extent be used as a prognostic marker. Recently, considerable insights into the epidemiology, pathology and genetics of the disease have been forthcoming, which should lead to a better definition of management strategies for women known to be harbouring germline mutations in predisposing genes.

Two genes have now been identified that are associated with familial clusterings of early-onset disease; however, evidence suggests the existence of additional predisposing genes (Sobol 1994; Rebeck et al. 1996; Serova et al. 1997; Kerangueven et al. 1995). Germline mutations in the BRCA1 gene predispose not only to breast cancer with a penetrance of 85% by 70 years of age but also ovarian cancer with a penetrance of approximately 40% by 70 years of age (Easton et al. 1994; Ford et al. 1995). Mutations in the BRCA2 gene predispose to breast cancer at similar rates to BRCA1, but are less

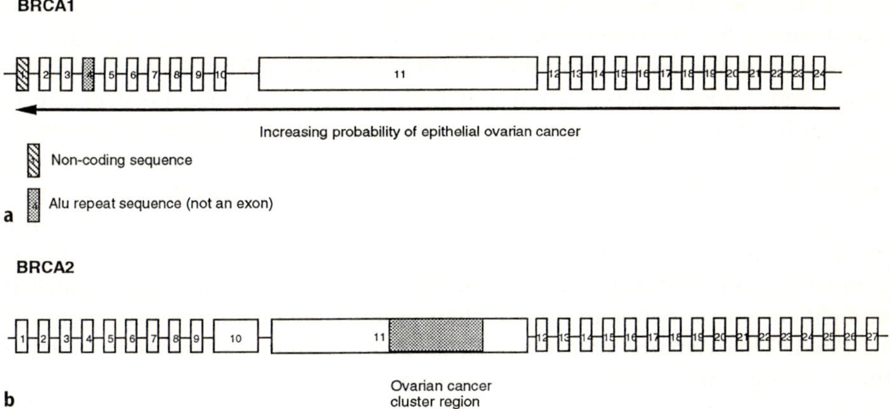

Fig. 2. Schematic representations of the **a** BRCA 1 and **b** BRCA 2 genes, indicating possible genotype/phenotype relationships. *Numbers* within the *boxes* indicate exon number (size not to scale)

likely to predispose to ovarian cancer (Ford and Easton 1995). Ovarian cancer penetrance in BRCA 2-linked families is approximately 27% by age 70 years (Easton 1997). In addition, breast cancer families harbour variable clinical presentations, potentially in relation to distinct molecular defects. Genotype–phenotype correlations have been reported concerning the tumour spectrum in BRCA 1-linked families, such that a gradient of likelihood (see Fig. 2 a) for ovarian cancer has been reported (Gayther et al. 1995). In BRCA 2-linked families an ovarian cancer cluster region (Fig. 2 b) has also been described (Gayther et al. 1996). The proliferation rate of tumours has also been shown to be increased (Sobol et al. 1996), and there are suggestions to indicate that disease penetrance may also be dependent on mutation site (Streuwing et al. 1997). If confirmed, these findings may help us to anticipate the occurrence of cancer and design prevention strategies as well as treatment for incident cancers in these families.

Evidence is accumulating that indicates that hereditary breast cancers harbour specific morphological patterns differentiating them from sporadic breast cancers (Jacquemier et al. 1995; Eisinger et al. 1996). In addition, pathologically there are differences between tumours derived from women harbouring BRCA 1 mutations and those harbouring BRCA 2 mutations (Marcus et al. 1996; Breast Cancer Linkage Consortium 1997). Medullary or atypical medullary tumours are more often present in BRCA 1-associated illness than in BRCA-2 linked illness, BRCA 2 tumours do not appear to have tubular carcinoma, and there is a lower incidence of this type of carcinoma in BRCA 1 tumours than in sporadic tumours. The grade of tumours resulting from both BRCA 1- and BRCA 2-associated cancers is significantly higher than that of controls, with higher mitosis rates and pleomorphism (Eisinger et al. 1996). Tubule formation is higher in BRCA 1 tumours than in BRCA 2 tumours (Breast Cancer Linkage Consortium 1997). In addition, a higher

Table 1. Classification of benign breast disease
(*RR* relative risk)

Nonproliferative – no increase in risk
  Cysts, micro or macro
  Duct ectasia
  Fibroadenoma
  Mastitis
  Fibrosis
  Metaplasia, squamous or apocrine
  Mild hyperplasia
Proliferative – RR 1.5–2.0
  Papilloma
  Sclerosing adenosis
  Hyperplasia, moderate or severe
Proliferative with atypia – RR 4.5–5.0
  Atypical ductal hyperplasia
  Atypical lobular hyperplasia

associated with no increase in the risk of breast cancer development, while proliferative lesions without atypia are associated with a small increase in breast cancer risk (RR 1.5–2.0). The greatest risk of breast cancer development (RR 4.0–5.0) is seen with atypical hyperplasia (Dupont and Page 1985). However, the absolute risk of breast cancer development 15 years after a diagnosis of atypical hyperplasia is only 8% in the absence of a family history of breast cancer. Approximately 70% of palpable breast masses contain nonproliferative disease (Dupont and Page 1985), and only 3.6% are atypical hyperplasia. The incidence of atypia is somewhat higher in biopsies performed for mammographic lesions, ranging from 7% to 10% (Morrow 1990; Rubin et al. 1988). Proliferative breast disease is also noted more frequently in women with a significant family history of breast cancer than in controls, further supporting its role as a risk factor (Skolnick et al. 1980).

Another benign breast lesion, which clearly is associated with an increased risk of breast cancer development, is lobular carcinoma in situ (LCIS). In the past LCIS was thought to be a malignant lesion, albeit one with a favorable prognosis. However, the finding that LCIS is associated with a risk of breast cancer development of approximately 1% per year, the observation that the risk of carcinoma is equal in both breasts, and the finding that neither the extent of LCIS in the breast nor its presence at a margin of resection influences the risk of subsequent cancer has led LCIS to be regarded as a risk factor for breast cancer development rather than the actual precursor of carcinoma (Morrow and Schnitt 1996). The reported incidence and relative risk of carcinoma in patients with LCIS are summarized in Table 2.

While LCIS is accepted as a breast cancer risk factor, ductal carcinoma in situ (DCIS) is usually considered to be an early cancer. The increased use of screening mammography has resulted in a marked increase in the detection rate of DCIS, as well as the recognition that the term DCIS encompasses a spectrum of disease entities. Low-grade DCIS lesions share many of the char-

Table 2. Risk of invasive carcinoma after lobular carcinoma in situ

Reference	Cases	% Invasive cancer	Relative risk
Haagensen et al. (1981)	287	18.0	6.9
Rosen et al. (1978)	99	34.5	9.0
Andersen (1974)	47	26.4	12.0
Page et al. (1991)	44	23.0	9.0
Salvadori et al. (1991)	80	6.3	10.0
Ottesen et al. (1993)	69	11.6	11.0

acteristics of LCIS, including a low proliferative rate, the presence of estrogen and progesterone receptors, and the absence of overexpression of p53 or C-erbB-2 protein (Porter et al. 1991; Bobrow et al. 1994; Zafrani et al. 1994). The relative risk of invasive carcinoma in a group of 25 women with DCIS initially misdiagnosed as having benign breast disease and treated by excision alone was 8 after 24 years of follow-up (Page et al. 1995), a level of risk very similar to that reported after a diagnosis of LCIS. The similarity in the biologic characteristics of LCIS and low-grade DCIS, as well as the similar risk of development of invasive carcinoma support the contention that some women with DCIS should be considered "high risk," rather than stage 0 cancer patients.

Environmental Factors and Diet

Exposure to ionizing radiation, whether secondary to nuclear explosion or to medical procedures, has been clearly demonstrated to increase breast cancer risk (Land and McGregor 1979; Hildreth et al. 1989; Miller et al. 1989; Hancock et al. 1993). The level of risk varies with the age at exposure, with a minimal increase in risk observed for exposures in women older than 40 years. Electromagnetic and solar radiation exposures have also been suggested to influence breast cancer risk (Loomis et al. 1994; Garland et al. 1990), but their role remains largely speculative. Organochlorines have been proposed as risk factors (Wolff et al. 1993), but further studies to confirm this association are needed.

A large amount of attention has been directed towards the role of diet in the etiology of breast cancer. This link has been suggested by the large international variation in breast cancer incidence rates and the observation that national per capita fat consumption correlates with breast cancer incidence and mortality. However, prospective studies of diet and breast cancer risk have failed to identify a relationship between dietary fat intake and breast cancer incidence for up to 10 years of follow-up (Hunter and Willett 1996). In the largest single prospective study to date, the Nurses Health Study, 89494 women were followed for 8 years, and 1439 developed breast carcinoma. The relative risk of cancer development among women in the highest quartile of fat intake was 0.86 (95% CI, 0.67–1.08) relative to women with the

Table 3. Magnitude of known breast cancer risk factors

Relative risk <2	Relative risk 2–4	Relative risk >4
Early menarche	Age >35 first birth	Gene mutations
Late menopause	1st-degree relative with breast cancer	Lobular carcinoma in situ
Nulliparity	Radiation exposure	Ductal carcinoma in situ
Proliferative benign disease	Prior breast cancer	Atypical hyperplasia
Obesity		
Alcohol use		
Hormone replacement		

lowest level of fat intake (Willett et al. 1992). The lack of a relationship between dietary fat intake and cancer risk within the context of a Western diet is confirmed by a pooled analysis of seven cohort studies involving a total of 337 819 women, which demonstrated no difference in risk for women in the lowest and highest quintiles for fat intake (Hunter et al. 1996). However, all of these studies have addressed fat intake in adult life, and they do not exclude the possibility that fat intake during childhood and adolescence may influence subsequent breast cancer risk.

Stronger evidence exists to support an association between alcohol and breast cancer. A meta-analysis of 12 case control studies demonstrated a relative risk of 1.4 for each 24 g of alcohol consumed daily (Longnecker et al. 1988). Defining a relationship between age of alcohol consumption and breast cancer risk is more difficult, with conflicting data on the importance of drinking early in life (Young 1989; Gapstur et al. 1992).

Summary of Risk Factors

In summary, although extensive studies of breast cancer risk factors have been carried out, many of the proposed associations remain unproven. Factors such as proliferative breast disease or nulliparity, which have clearly been proven to increase risk in studies of large populations have little measing for the individual woman owing to the small increased increment in risk which they convey. A classification of risk factors as major or minor, and the relative risk associated with these factors is shown in Table 3.

Interactions Among Risk Factors

A major problem in the clinical identification of the "high-risk woman" is the lack of knowledge of the interactions among the various factors known to alter breast cancer risk, since the majority of studies have focused on defining individual risk factors. Most women have a combination of factors that both increase risk and are protective, complicating the assessment of an individual's level of risk. In addition, it is unclear whether the risk conferred by multiple risk factors is additive, multiplicative, or varies with the risk factor under study.

The interactions between the family history of breast cancer and other risk factors have been examined, often with conflicting results. Dupont and Page (1985) observed that the combination of atypical hyperplasia and a family history of a first-degree relative with breast cancer increased the relative risk of breast cancer to 11 times that of an index population, as against a relative risk of 4.4 for atypia alone. However, Rosen et al. (1978) found that the presence of a family history of breast carcinoma did not alter the level of risk after a diagnosis of lobular carcinoma in situ, a lesion often considered part of a continuum with atypical hyperplasia. An analysis of data from the Nurses Health Study (Colditz et al. 1993) showed that in women with a mother or sister with breast cancer, known risk factors relating to age at menarche or menopause, parity, age at first birth, alcohol use, and the presence of benign breast disease did not further alter risk. In contrast, Anderson and Badzioch (1989) and Brinton et al. (1982) have reported that hormonal factors modulate risk further in women with a family history of breast cancer, although the effect varies with the factor under study.

Studies of the interaction between estrogen replacement therapy and other known breast cancer risk factors also have variable results, depending on the risk factor under study. In a meta-analysis of 16 published studies, Steinberg et al. (1991) found that the effect of estrogen replacement did not differ among parous and nulliparous women and those with or without benign breast disease. However, an enhanced risk was observed in women with a family history of breast cancer.

The analysis of the interaction among risk factors is further complicated by the fact that some factors may be important for the risk of premenopausal, but not postmenopausal, cancer and vice versa, and these effects may not be constant over time. For example, long duration of lactation appears to reduce premenopausal breast cancer risk, but has little impact on the risk of the more frequently encountered postmenopausel breast cancer (Newcomb et al. 1994). Pregnancy in general reduces breast cancer risk, but for a short period following pregnancy risk is actually increased (Lambe et al. 1994). Women with proliferative breast disease have a doubling of their relative risk of breast cancer, but 10 years after diagnosis this risk returns to baseline. Similarly, the relative risk seen with a diagnosis of atypical hyperplasia is halved after a 10-year interval (Dupont and Page 1989).

A model to predict the risk of breast cancer development in women at a given age over a defined time interval was developed by Gail et al. (1989) using data from 4,496 matched pairs of cases and controls in the Breast Cancer Diagnosis and Demonstration Project. The model incorporates the risk factors of age at menarche, age at first live birth, number of first-degree relatives with breast cancer, and number of previous breast biopsies, and has been shown to predict risk accurately in two validation studies of women undergoing annual mammographic screening (Bondy et al. 1994; Spiegelman et al. 1994). However, the model overpredicts breast cancer risk by 33% among women aged 60 and younger who do not undergo annual screening. There are several other limitations of the model. Because only first-degree relatives are considered, it is not an appropriate model for women with extensive family histories of breast cancer, whose risk may be underestimated. In women with risk due to lobular carcinoma in situ, ductal carcinoma in situ, or atypical hyperplasia, the model unterestimates risk, since the highest relative risk for breast biopsy is 2.0. Similarly, for the woman with non-proliferative disease, the model may overestimate risk. In spite of these limitations, the model is a clinically useful tool for identifying a woman's level of risk over a clinically relevant time period, after correction for competing causes of mortality.

Definition of a "High-Risk" Population

From the preceding discussion, it can be appreciated that the problem of identification of the high-risk women is far from solved. Many "risk factors" lack firm documentation of their clinical significance, and the interaction among risk factors and their variability over time are poorly understood. The vast majority of data on risk come from studies of white women, and little is known about the impact of ethnic diversity on the importance of these factors. In addition, there is no consensus regarding what level of increase in risk is necessary for a woman to a labeled "high risk." It is noteworthy that even among women with the risk factors associated with the highest risk of breast cancer development, the majority will not develop breast carcinoma. Great caution must be exercised in labeling a women as high risk, since such a label often results in increased anxiety for both the woman and her physician, with the potential for excessive numbers of mammograms and breast biopsies.

Definition of a high-risk population is relevant only when an effective and acceptable intervention to reduce risk is available. As breast cancer prevention becomes a clinical reality (see chapters by Jordan and by Powles in this volume), it is appropriate to question whether prevention strategies that target high-risk women are likely to have a major impact on the problem of breast cancer mortality. A recent study of the fraction of breast cancer cases in the United States attributable to well-established risk factors identified only 47% of patients as having attributable risk factors (Madigan et al. 1995). A family history of breast cancer accounted for only 9.1% of cases, while relatively minor risk factors, such as later age at first birth and nulliparity, contributed 29.5% of cases. In a similar study, Seidman et al. (1982) noted that only 21% of breast cancer cases in women aged 30–54 and 29% of cases in women aged 55–84 occurred in women with 1 of 10 common breast cancer risk factors. The majority of women in the studies described had minor risk factors that increase the relative risk of breast cancer only two-fold, and most had only a single risk factor. This level of "increased risk" would not meet the entry criteria for the ongoing trials of breast cancer prevention.

These date suggest that even if women with a very small increase in breast cancer risk were targeted for prevention initiatives, a large number of cases would continue to be missed. Prevention strategies which are applicable to all women are needed until our understanding of the pathogenesis of breast cancer allows a more accurate definition of what constitutes a high-risk woman.

References

Anderson DE, Badzioch MD (1989) Combined effect of family history and reproductive factors on breast cancer risk. Cancer 63:349–353

Anderson JA (1984) Lobular carcinoma in situ. A long term follow-up in 52 cases. Acta Pathol Microbiol Scand 85:519–533

Bernstein L, Henderson BE, Hanisch R et al (1994) Physical exercise activity reduces the risk of breast cancer in young women. J Natl Cancer Inst 86:1403–1408

Bobrow LG, Happerfield LC, Gregory WM et al (1994) The classification of ductal carcinoma in situ and its association with biological markers. Semin Diagn Pathol 11:199–207

Bondy M, Lustbader ED, Halabi S et al (1994) Validation of a breast cancer risk assessment model in women with a positive family history. J Natl Cancer Inst 86:620–625

Brinton L, William R, Hoover R et al (1979) Breast cancer risk factors among screening program participants. J Natl Cancer Inst 62:37–44

Brinton LA, Hoover R, Fraumeni JF (1982) Interaction of familial and hormonal risk factors for breast cancer. J Natl Cancer Inst 69:817–822

Colditz GA, Willett WC, Hunter DJ et al (1993) Family history, age, and risk of breast cancer. Prospective data from the Nurses' Healthy study. JAMA 270:338–343

Daling JR, Malone KE, Voight LF, White E, Weiss NS (1994) Risk of breast cancer among young women: relationship to induced abortion. J Natl Cancer Inst 86:1584–1592

Dewaard F, Baanders-van Halewijn E (1974) A prospective study in general practice on breast cancer risk in postmenopausal women. Int J Cancer 14:153–160

Dorgan JF, Brown C, Barrett M et al (1994) Physical activity and risk of breast cancer in the Framingham heart study. Am J Epidemiol 139:662–669

Duffy S, Robert M, Elton R (1983) Risk factors for breast cancer: relevance to screening. J Epidemiol Community Health 37:127–131

Dupont WD, Page D (1985) Risk factors for breast cancer in women with proliferative breast disease. N Engl J Med 312:146–151

Dupont WD, Page D (1989) Relative risk of breast cancer varies with time since diagnosis of atypical hyperplasia. Hum Pathol 20:723–725

Ekbom A, Trichopoulos D, Adami H et al (1995) Evidence of prenatal influence on breast cancer risk. Lancet 340:1015–1018

Frisch R, Gotz-Welbergen A, McArthur J et al (1981) Delayed menarche and amenorrhea of college athletes in relation to age of onset of training. JAMA 246:1559–1563

Gail MH, Brinton LA, Byar DP et al (1989) Projecting individualized probabilities of developing breast cancer for white females who are being examined annually. J Natl Cancer Inst 81:1879–1886

Gapstur SM, Potter JD, Folsom AR (1992) Increased risk of breast cancer with alcohol consumption in postmenopausal women. Am J Epidemiol 136:1221–1231

Garland FC, Garland CF, Gorham ED et al (1990) Geographic variation in breast cancer mortality in the United States: a hypothesis involving exposure to solar radiation. Prev Med 19:614–622

Haagensen CD, Bodian C, Haagensen DE (1981) Lobular neoplasia (lobular carcinoma in situ). In: Haagensen CD, Bodian C, Haagensen DE (eds) Breast carcinoma: risk and detection. Saunders, Philadelphia

Hancock SL, Tucker MA, Hoppe RT (1993) Breast cancer after treatment of Hodgkin's disease. J Natl Cancer Inst 85:25–31

Harris BM, Eklund G, Meirik O, Rutqvist LE, Wiklund L (1989) Risk of cancer of the breast after legal abortion during the first trimester: a Swedish register study. BMJ 299:1430–1432

Henderson B, Ross R, Bernstein L (1988) Estrogens as a cause of human cancer: the Richard and Hinda Rosenthal Foundation Award Lecture. Cancer Res 48:246–253

Hildreth NG, Shore RE, Dvoretsky PM (1989) The risk of breast cancer after irradiation of the thymus in infancy. N Engl J Med 321:1281–1284

Hunter D, Spiegelman D, Adami H et al (1996) Cohort studies of fat intake and the risk of breast cancer: a pooled analysis. N Engl J Med 334:356–361

Hunter DJ, Willett WC (1996) Dietary factors. In: Harris JR, Lippman ME, Morrow M, Hellman S (eds) Disease of the Breast. Lippincott-Raven, Philadelphia, pp 201–212

Hutter R (1986) Consensus meeting: Is "fibrocystic disease" of the breast precancerous? Arch Pathol Lab Med 110:171–173

Kvale G, Heuch I (1988) Lactation and cancer risk: is there a relation specific to breast cancer? J Epidemiol Community Health 42:30–37

Lambe M, Hsieh CC, Trichopoulos D et al (1994) Transient increase in the risk of breast cancer after giving birth. N Engl J Med 331:5–12

Land CE, McGregor DH (1979) Breast cancer incidence among atomic bomb survivors: implications for radiobiologic risk at low doses. J Natl Cancer Inst 62:17–21

Layde PM, Webster LA, Baughman AL (1989) The independent associations of parity, age at first full-term pregnancy, and duration of breast feeding with the risk of breast cancer. J Clin Epidemiol 42:963–973

London SJ, Colditz GA, Stampfer WJ et al (1989) Prospective study of relative weight, height, and risk of breast cancer. JAMA 262:2853–2858

Longnecker M, Berlin J, Orza M et al (1988) A metaanalysis of alcohol consumption in relation to breast cancer risk. JAMA 260:652–656

Loomis DP, Savitz DA, Ananth CV (1994) Breast cancer mortality among female electrical workers in the United States. J Natl Cancer Inst 86:921–925

MacMahon B, Cole P, Lin T (1970) Age at first birth and breast cancer risk. Bull WHO 43:209–210

MacMahon B, Trichopoulos D, Brown J et al (1982) Age at menarche, probability of ovulation and breast cancer risk. Int J Cancer 298:13–16

Madigan MP, Ziegler RG, Benichou J et al (1995) Proportion of breast cancer cases in the United States explained by well-established risk factors. J Natl Cancer Inst 87:1681–1685

Malone KE, Daling JR, Weiss N (1993) Oral contraception in relation to breast cancer. Epidemiol Rev 15:80–97

Meirik O, Lunde E, Adami H et al (1986) Oral contraceptive use and breast cancer in younger women. A joint national case control study in Sweden and Norway. Lancet II:650–654

Melbye M, Wohlfohrt J, Olsen JH et al (1997) Induced abortion and the risk of breast cancer. N Engl J Med 336:81–85

Miller AB, Howe GR, Sherman GJ et al (1989) Mortality from breast cancer after irradiation during fluoroscopic examinations in patients being treated for tuberculosis. N Engl J Med 321:1285–1298

Morrow M (1990) Management of nonpalpable breast masses. PPO Updates 4:1–11

Morrow M (1992) Pre-cancerous breast lesions: implications for breast cancer prevention trials. Int J Radiat Oncol Biol Phys 23:1071–1078

Morrow M, Schnitt SJ (1996) Lobular carcinoma in situ. In: Harris JR, Lippman ME, Morrow M, Hellman S (eds) Diseases of the breast. Lippincott-Raven, Philadelphia, pp 369–374

Newcomb PA, Storer BE, Longnecker MP et al (1994) Lactation and a reduced risk of premenopausal breast cancer. N Engl J Med 330:81–87

Newcomb PA, Storer BE, Longnecker MP, Mittendorf R, Greenberg ER, Willett WC (1996) Pregnancy termination in relation to risk of breast cancer. JAMA 275:283–287

Ottesen GL, Graversen HP, Blichert-Tort M et al (1993) Lobular carcinoma in situ of the female breast. Short-term results of a prospective nationwide study. Am J Surg Pathol 17:14–21

Page DL, Kidd TE, Dupont WD et al (1991) Lobular neoplasia of the breast: higher risk for subsequent invasive cancer predicted by more extensive disease. Hum Pathol 22:1232–1239

Page DL, Dupont WD, Rogers LW et al (1995) Continued local recurrence of carcinoma 15–25 years after a diagnosis of low grade ductal carcinoma in situ of the breast treated only by biopsy. Cancer 76:1197–1200

Porter BL, Garcia R, Moe R et al (1991) C-erb-2 oncogene protein in situ and invasive lobular breast neoplasia. Cancer 68:331–334

Ries LAG, Miller BA, Hankey BF et al (eds) (1994) SEER Cancer Statistics Review, 1973–1991. (NIH publication 94–2789) US DHHS National Cancer Institute, Bethesda

Rosen PP, Lieberman PH, Braun DW Jr et al (1978) Lobular carcinoma in situ of the breast. Am J Surg Pathol 2:225–251

Rubin E, Visscher D, Alexander R et al (1988) Proliferative disease and atypia in biopsies performed for nonpalpable lesions detected mammographically. Cancer 61:2077–2082

Salvadori B, Bartoli C, Zurrida S et al (1991) Risk of invasive cancer in women with lobular carcinoma in situ of the breast. Eur J Cancer 27:35–37

Seidman H, Stellman SD, Mushinski MH (1982) A different perspective on breast cancer risk factors: some implications of non-attributable risk. CA Cancer J Clin 32:301–312

Sillero-Arenas M, Delgado-Rodriguez M, Rodigues-Canteras R et al (1992) Menopausal hormone replacement therapy and breast cancer: a meta-analysis. Obstet Gynecol 79:286–294

Skolnick M, Cannon-Albright L, Goldgar D et al (1990) Inheritance of proliferative breast disease in breast cancer kindreds. Science 250:1715–1720

Spiegelman D, Colditz GA, Hunter D et al (1994) Validation of the Gail et al. model predicting individual breast cancer risk. J Natl Cancer Inst 86:600–607

Steinberg KK, Thacker SB, Smith J et al (1991) A meta-analysis of the effect of estrogen replacement therapy on the risk of breast cancer. JAMA 265:1985–1990

Trichopoulos D, MacMahon B, Cole P (1972) Menopause and breast cancer risk. J Natl Cancer Inst 48:605–613

UK National Case-Control Study Group (1989) Oral contraceptive use and breast cancer risk in young women. Lancet I:976–982

Willett WC, Hunger DJ, Stampfer MJ et al (1992) Dietary fat and fiber in relation to risk of breast cancer. An 8 year follow-up. JAMA 268:2037–2044

Wolff MS, Toniolo PG, Lee EW et al (1993) Blood levels of organocholorine residues and risk of breast cancer. J Natl Cancer Inst 85:648–652

Young TB (1989) A case-control study of breast cancer and alcohol consumption habits. Cancer 64:552–558

Zafrani B, Leroyer A, Fourquet A et al (1994) Mammographically detected ductal in situ carcinoma of the breast analyzed with a new classification. A study of 127 cases: correlation with estrogen and progesterone receptors, p 53 and C-erb B-2 proteins, and proliferative activity. Semin Diagn Pathol 11:208–214

Development of a New Prevention Maintenance Therapy for Postmenopausal Women

V. Craig Jordan

Robert H. Lurie Cancer Center, Northwestern University Medical School, Chicago, IL 60611 USA

Abstract

In spring 1998, breast cancer prevention emerged from being a concept to being a reality. The National Surgical Adjuvant Breast and Bowel Project prevention trial showed that tamoxifen reduced breast cancer by 45% in high-risk women between the ages of 35 and 75. Additionally, an evaluation of 10 550 patients randomized to osteoporosis trials of placebo versus raloxifene demonstrated a 50% reduction in the incidence of breast cancer in woman taking raloxifene. For the future, a Study of Tamoxifen Against Raloxifene (STAR) is ongoing in high-risk postmenopausal women. This chapter describes the biological rationale for the current clinical advances.

Introduction

The success of public health initiatives and the development of vaccines and antibiotics have radically improved the welfare of society in the twentieth Century. However, our successes have created new problems that require solutions. Life expectancy has increased steadily, and, with an aging population, new challenges to control the progression of osteoporosis, coronary heart disease and breast cancer have become international priorities in the industrialized countries. Hormone replacement therapy with estrogen offers important benefits for the woman during and after the menopause. Most women who take Premarin, for example, use a short course of a year or two at the most, to ameliorate hot flashes and depression in their early fifties. However, it is now clear that long-term or perhaps lifetime estrogen replacement therapy is the best strategy to prevent osteoporosis and coronary heart disease. These two diseases alone are the major killers of women in their sixties and seventies, and the benefits of estrogen far outweigh the risks. Nevertheless, the principal concerns that often prevent women from embarking on a life-long course of hormone replacement therapy are the perceived increased risks of breast and endometrial cancer. Although periodic adminis-

Recent Results in Cancer Research, Vol. 151
Senn/Costa/Jordan (Eds.): Chemoprevention of Cancer
© Springer-Verlag Berlin · Heidelberg 1999

tration of a progestin for the appropriate duration can reduce concerns about endometrial cancer, a prevention strategy based on withdrawal bleeding is inconvenient. Additionally, progestins do not protect against breast cancer, and some have argued that there are slight increases in risk. Although there is much debate about whether hormone replacement therapy increases or does not affect the risk of breast cancer, this is not the point. Overall there is no decrease in breast cancer risk, and it is this observation that creates the dilemma.

During the 1990s there has been a fierce international debate about the appropriate measures, and research to prevent breast cancer. Women in their forties have been at the forefront as advocates, but the medical community is uncertain about recommendations because of a lack of knowledge. In the main this is because the time needed to prove prevention strategies often exceeds the life expectancy of the current generation of women and investigators! One approach is to employ current knowledge about effective treatments of breast cancer and design clinical trials to test the worth of a preventive strategy. This is the approach that has been taken with the antiestrogen tamoxifen.

We have known for a century that (1) estrogen withdrawal will prevent the continuing growth of some breast cancers (Beatson 1896; Boyd 1900) and (2) an oophorectomy in a woman's thirties will reduce the subsequent risk of breast cancer by 50%. Clearly the use of an antiestrogenic drug to prevent breast cancer in high-risk populations has scientific merit.

Tamoxifen has been used for the treatment of breast cancer for a quarter of a century (Jordan 1997a, b). The drug is now the endocrine treatment of choice for all stages of breast cancer and is listed by the World Health Organization as an essential cancer therapy. More than a million patients world wide are currently taking tamoxifen, and it is estimated that clinical experience draws on 9 million woman-years of use.

In 1986, Dr. Trevor Powles, at the Royal Marsden Hospital in England, initiated a vangard study to test the worth of tamoxifen as a preventive in high-risk women. The study was initiated on the basis of three emerging facts: (1) tamoxifen was well tolerated with a minimum of side effects (Furr and Jordan 1984); (2) tamoxifen prevents mammary carcinogenesis in rats (Jordan 1974, 1976); and (3) tamoxifen reduces the risk of contralateral breast cancer (Cuzick and Baum 1985). The goal was to randomize 2000 high-risk women to receive tamoxifen or placebo for 8 years and to evaluate compliance, toxicology and issues such as circulating cholesterol and bone density. These data have been garnered during the past decade (Powles et al. 1989, 1990, 1994, 1996), but in a parallel venture we proposed a broader strategy that could act as a prevention maintenance therapy in all postmenopausal women.

This chapter will trace the change in thinking about the prevention of breast cancer during the past quarter of a century. The story is the story of the development of tamoxifen. By a fortunate series of circumstance this is also the duration of tenure of Professor Hans-Jörge Senn at the Department of Oncology in St. Gallen. I dedicate this history to him, to celebrate his 25th anniversary and to acknowledge the immense prestige his contributions to clinical oncology have brought to St. Gallen and to Switzerland.

The Development of Tamoxifen

Twenty-five years ago (1972) there was not tamoxifen, but only an antiestrogen ICI 46474 with partial antiestrogenic activity and antifertility properties in laboratory animals (Harper and Walpole 1967a, b). Since it was realized that antiestrogens could be valuable therapeutic agents, the drug was evaluated for a number of clinical applications. Originally tamoxifen was marketed for the induction of ovulation in subfertile women, but because of modest activity in the palliation of advanced breast cancer (Cole et al. 1971; Ward 1973) it was introduced as an endocrine option for the treatment of advanced breast cancer in postmenopausal women in the United Kingdom in 1973 and in the United States in 1978. Although tamoxifen or Nolvadex was equally efficacious as other endocrine therapies at the time, there was a low reported incidence of side effects, which ultimately became extremely important for subsequent drug development.

During the 1970s adjuvant therapy regimens were tested internationally to find a cure for node-positive and subsequently node-negative breast cancer. Although numerous chemotherapeutic regimens were evaluated, singly and in combination, the endocrine therapy tested was tamoxifen. Initially, clinical trials had a 1-year duration, because tamoxifen was only effective for about 1 year in the treatment of advanced disease. Most importantly, though, there were sincere concerns that too long a duration of tamoxifen would prematurely precipitate tamoxifen-resistant disease and the value of the palliative agent would be lost as an option for the treatment of a recurrence (reviewed by Jordan 1994).

The successful development of tamoxifen is the result of a dialogue between laboratory scientists keen to develop reasonable treatment strategies and the clinical community's willingness to test the ideas in large randomized clinical trials. The optimal duration of adjuvant tamoxifen therapy is a case in point. In 1977, at a breast cancer symposium in Cambridge, England (see Jordan 1997a, b), we demonstrated that long-term, perhaps indefinite, tamoxifen therapy would be necessary to provide optimal effects. We proposed that tamoxifen exhibited the properties of a tumoristatic agent, so that continuous therapy was necessary to control the estrogen-stimulated growth of micrometastatic disease. All the studies of 1 year of tamoxifen failed to demonstrate survival advantages, but the principle that longer could be better was illustrated by the subsequent results of the NATO (Nolvadex Adjuvant Trial Organization 1985) and Scottish Trials (Breast Cancer Trials Committee, Scottish Trials Office 1987), which demonstrated that 2 or 5 years of adjuvant tamoxifen would confer a survival advantage. Today it is known that 5 years is superior to 2 years of tamoxifen (Swedish Breast Cancer Cooperative

Group 1996), but there is still controversy about the optimal duration of adjuvant tamoxifen. Although the results of an estrogen receptor (ER)-positive node-negative breast cancer trial in pre- and postmenopausal women demonstrated that continuing tamoxifen past 5 years provided no further benefit (Fisher et al. 1996), there is no general agreement that this is the final word on duration. Professor Richard Peto at Oxford has argued (Peto 1996) that larger clinical trials are necessary to prove the point for all stages of breast cancer. As a result, the ATLAS (Adjuvant Tamoxifen Long Against Short) and the aTTom (adjuvant Tamoxifen Treatment offer more) clinical trials, both based in the United Kingdom, are each recruiting 20000 patients to either stop or continue tamoxifen for another 5 years at whatever point they are currently being treated i.e.: 5, 8, 10 years, etc. The large data base, and the assessment of toxicology, will define both efficacy and patient acceptability.

Overall the ubiquitous use of tamoxifen has revolutionized the treatment of all stages of breast cancer. The general adoption of a strategy of long-term tamoxifen treatment by the mid-1980s did, however, produce a new set of concerns. If patients with node-negative disease were to be treated for up to a decade with an antiestrogen would this produce other physiologic problems? Estrogen is essential to maintain bone density and to maintain a beneficial profile of circulating lipids. Would long-term antiestrogen therapy predispose patients cured of breast cancer to osteoporosis and coronary heart disease?

Target-site-specific Effects of Antiestrogens

Concerns about the long-term safety of tamoxifen prompted an investigation into its effects on bone density and circulating lipids. Without these studies it was clear that the testing of tamoxifen as a preventive in high-risk women could not be attempted safely, and truly undesirable findings would restrict the use of tamoxifen as a treatment. It would be unwise, for example, to treat low risk node-negative women with a drug that increased the risk of coronary heart disease and osteoporosis.

During the mid-1980s we published the results from a series of pivotal laboratory studies that would ultimately define the strategy to develop a postmenopausal prevention maintenance therapy (Jordan et al. 1987; Gottardis and Jordan 1987; Gottardis et al. 1988). However, although the ultimate goal was the wide therapeutic use of targeted antiestrogens, the immediate aim was to address issues surrounding tamoxifen. There was a focused desire to test tamoxifen as a breast cancer preventive, so all the relevant research was centered on the only drug available for clinical testing. Nevertheless, the principles are now clear and the results can be translated for the evaluation of any new agent.

In the laboratory we found that tamoxifen and, a then relatively unknown drug, keoxifene (now known as raloxifene) maintain bone density in ovariectomized rats. Indeed, estrogen plus the antiestrogens had an additive effect on bone, but the drugs inhibited the action of estrogen on the uterus. The work illustrated the target-site-specific actions of antiestrogens and demonstrated the potential of an antiestrogen to switch on or switch off different sites around a woman's body (Jordan et al. 1987) We concluded:

The mechanism of the disparate pharmacology is unknown, but these results may have important implication for the clinical applications of antiestrogens. Estrogen is used for the prevention of osteoporosis in postmenopausal women. Early concerns about an increased risk of developing endometrial carcinoma have been ameliorated by the sequential use of oral progestational agents followed by steroid withdrawal to precipitate menses. It is possible however, that in the future tamoxifen could be considered to be used as a substitute estrogen in this setting. This could serve a dual purpose: to further reduce the risk of endometrial carcinoma because the drug has been used to treat the disease, and potentially to reduce the risk of developing breast cancer, while still preventing bone density loss. (Jordan et al. 1987)

We successfully translated these data to a clinical trial to demonstrate that an antiestrogen can maintain bone density in postmenopausal women (Love et al. 1992). Today our results have been adequately confirmed (Kristensen et al. 1994; Ward et al. 1993), and the concept is the basis of the current interest in developing target-site-specific drugs to prevent osteoporosis (Tonetti and Jordan 1996; Jordan 1997c).

As a side issue, the data monitoring committee of the Wisconsin Tamoxifen Study chose to measure circulating cholesterol and other risk factors for cardiovascular disease in our double blind randomized clinical trial monitoring bone density. There had already been sporadic case reports that tamoxifen lowered cholesterol, but our large clinical trial established that although tamoxifen lowers total circulating cholesterol only the low-density lipoprotein (LDL) cholesterol component is decreased (Love et al. 1991). High-density lipoprotein cholesterol remains unaffected. These effects may be partly responsible for the decreases in coronary heart disease (McDonald and Stewart 1992; McDonald et al. 1995; Costantino et al. 1997) or hospital visits for any cardiac condition (Rutqvist and Matteson 1993) noted in patients taking tamoxifen. Indeed, there is a suggestion from these data that longer term therapy might provide better protection from coronary heart disease in high-risk populations (Jordan 1997c).

Thus, the pieces were in place to test tamoxifen as a preventive. However, not all the news was good. We noted that tamoxifen could encourage the growth of pre-existing endometrial cancer (Gottardis et al. 1988). We alerted the clinical community, but our call, unfortunately, resulted in an overreaction to the problem. Fortunately the extent of the problem can now be placed in perspective.

The Endometrial Cancer Controversy

In 1988 we completed a series of laboratory experiments to illustrate the target site specificity of tamoxifen in breast and endometrial cancer. We found that if athymic mice were bitransplanted with a breast and an endometrial tumor and then the animals were treated with both estrogen and tamoxifen, the drug would prevent estrogen-stimulated breast cancer growth but endometrial cancer growth was stimulated (Gottardis et al. 1988). Although endometrial cancer had been noted in three patients with breast cancer treated with tamoxifen (Killacky et al. 1985) this was not surprising, as there is a known association between breast and endometrial cancer and indeed tamoxifen had been used to treat endometrial cancer, so that the clinical disease extent could really have been controlled by the drug. The unique feature of our report was the fact that the estrogen-stimulated growth of breast, but not endometrial cancer, could be controlled by tamoxifen. We therefore called for a closer examination of patients during tamoxifen treatment. We wrote:

> Endometrial carcinoma has been reported to develop during tamoxifen therapy. However the fact that tamoxifen has been successfully used to treat endometrial cancer does not exclude the possibility of an increasing incidence of endometrial tumors during prolonged tamoxifen therapy for breast cancer. A larger cohort of patients under long-term tamoxifen therapy (>5 years) needs to be monitored for the occurrence of tamoxifen stimulated endometrial tumors. (Gottardis et al. 1988)

In response, the clinical community rapidly started to document the association between tamoxifen and endometrial cancer (Hardel 1988; Fornander et al. 1989). The Stockholm group actually demonstrated the target site specificity of tamoxifen in their cohort of patients: contralateral breast cancer was decreased but the incidence of endometrial cancer was increased.

Although there were initial concerns that tamoxifen would cause an unacceptable increase in endometrial cancer and that this disease would be aggressive and of a grade to involve a poor prognosis (Magriples et al. 1993), this is not the case. We have routinely surveyed the world literature to define the extent of the association between tamoxifen and endometrial cancer, and it is modest (Assikis et al. 1996). At most there is a twofold increase in risk, and the disease has the same stage and grade as in the general population. Indeed this would be expected, as there is known to be a fourfold excess of occult disease compared to clinically detected disease (Horwitz and Feinstein 1986). Since tamoxifen can produce symptoms such as vaginal discharge, this will lead to increased screening of women taking tamoxifen, so naturally occult disease will be discovered.

The international concern about tamoxifen prompted the International Agency for Reserach on Cancer, a subgroup of the World Health Organization, to review the links between tamoxifen and carcinogenesis. They found there was an association between tamoxifen and endometrial cancer, but the committee stated that no woman should stop taking tamoxifen for the treatment of breast cancer on the basis of its conclusions. The benefits of tamoxifen far outweigh the risks. Be that as it may, the issue of carcinogenesis is extremely important when the introduction of a new drug for the general population as a prevention maintenance therapy or preventive for osteoporosis is considered. Without knowledge derived in the laboratory, and with the findings of the preliminary clinical studies (Hardel 1988; Fornander et al. 1989) that confirmed our laboratory concerns (Gottardis et al. 1988), we changed the focus of our strategy away from tamoxifen (Lerner and Jordan 1990). We wrote:

Important clues have been garnered about the effects of tamoxifen on bone and lipids, so it is possible that derivatives could find targeted applications to retard osteoporosis or atherosclerosis. The ubiquitous application of novel compounds to prevent diseases associated with progressive changes after the menopause may, as a side effect, significantly retard the development of breast cancer. The targeted population would be post menopausal women in general thereby avoiding the requirement to select a high risk group to prevent breast cancer.

Clearly this left raloxifene for drug development.

A Prevention Strategy for Breast Cancer

Despite the concerns expressed by pressure groups about the safety of tamoxifen, three separate clinical trials started in the early 1990s to test the worth of tamoxifen as a preventive. There is no doubt that the concerns were overstated and the trials went ahead based exclusively on the fact that clinical experience demonstrated tamoxifen's safety; an overview of trials showed that tamoxifen reduces the incidence of contralateral breast cancer by 38% (Early Breast Cancer Trialist Collaborative Group 1992). The current status of the trials will be explained briefly. In the United States the National Surgical Adjuvant Breast and Bowel Project has now (Summer, 1991) completed recruitment to a two-arm study comparing tamoxifen (20 mg daily) with placebo (Fig. 1). Thirteen thousand high-risk women have been randomized to receive treatments for 5 years. In the United Kingdom, the vanguard study initiated by Dr. Trevor Powles is now complete (see his chapter in this volume), and an international study has been opened up to general recruitment in a 20 000 volunteer trial. Finally, in Italy women volunteers over the age of 45 who have already had a hysterectomy are being recruited to a 20 000 volunteer trial. Overall these trials will offer enormous insight into the value of tamoxifen as a preventive and the safety of the modality. However, the requirement to evaluate high-risk women for the trial in the United States and the United Kingdom may ultimately be too narrow a focus to have a significant impact on public health nationally.

There is currently enormous interest in the application predisposing factors to predict the risks for breast cancer. This topic is considered in depth by Dr. Monica Morrow in this volume; however, the reports by Madigan et al. (1995) and Vogel (1996) on the analysis of risks factors and the subsequent development of breast cancer are particularly instructive. Overall, the known risk factors account for approximately half of the breast cancers. An example is illustrated in Fig. 2. The good news is that a women with risk factors can be monitored closely, but the bad news is that breast cancer occurs, half the time, in women without any risk factors. Clearly a pro-active strategy for breast cancer prevention needs to be put in place. At present there is

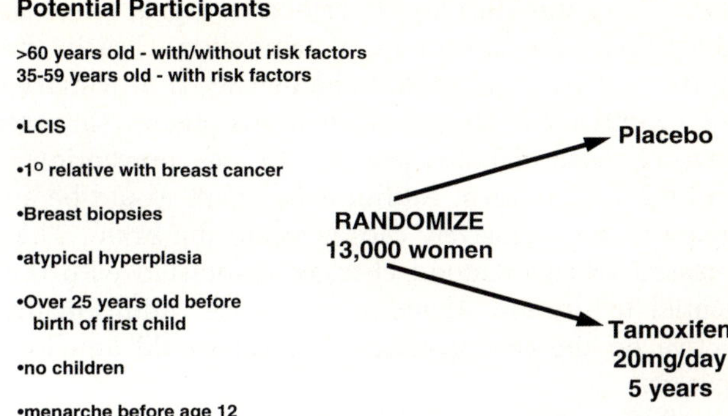

Fig. 1. Schema of entry requirements to the NSABP prevention trial in North America. High-risk women (estimated to be at least RR=4 for each age group) have been randomized to receive tamoxifen, a single dose of 20 mg daily, or placebo for 5 years. Originally 16000 volunteers were to be recruited, but the re-evaluation of risk showed that the actual risk estimate of volunteers was higher than originally projected. As a result, the recruitment goal was reduced

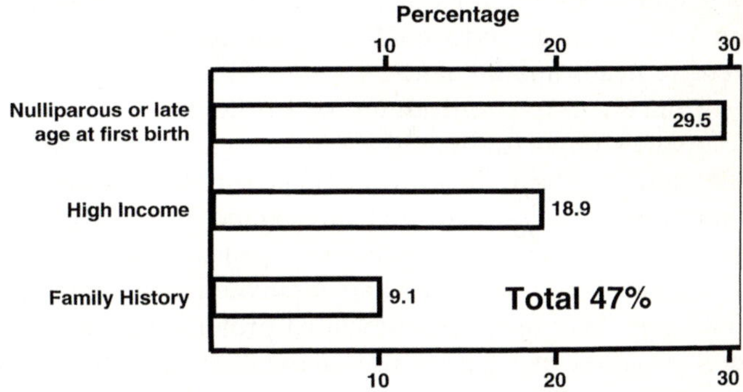

Fig. 2. Population-attributable risk of breast cancer based on three known risk factors in a series of breast cancer patients (Madigan et al. 1995). Although 47% of cases could be accounted for by these known risk factors, the majority of women did not carry the risk factors

no scientifically based intervention, other than close monitoring, that can be employed by a physician to aid patients. Before a description of a potential solution to this public health dilemma, it is appropriate to consider the scientific rationale for the design of a targeted antiestrogen as a prevention maintenance therapy.

An Ideal Targeted Antiestrogen

The expanding database concerning the toxicology and biological effects of antiestrogens presents the opportunity to design an agent with idea properties. These qualities are described in Fig. 3, based upon our experiences with the clinical pharmacology of tamoxifen. Clearly the target site specificity of antiestrogens to preserve bone density is a primary quality that has provided an incentive for clinical drug development. However, the ability to decrease LDL cholesterol holds promise for the prevention of coronary heart disease in high-risk women. Additionally, there would be an advantage for a targeted agent to be exclusively estrogenic in the brain. The advantages would be expressed as fewer mood changes associated with the menopause and the potential to prevent Alzheimer's disease. Additionally, estrogen-like properties active on the cardiovascular system would ameliorate hot flashes and night sweats.

All the above qualities can be met effectively by estrogen preparations and, as mentioned in the Introduction, the value of estrogen replacement, on balance, for women's health has been validated in numerous studies. However, for the millions of postmenopausal women who wish to embark on a prevention strategy, perhaps for decades, a targeted antiestrogen or designer estrogen is required to be an antiestrogen in the breast and uterus to prevent the promotional action of endogenous estrogen. The new agent would be invaluable to the millions of women who are concerned about their risk factors for breast cancer and would allow the physician to offer a new option in preventive health maintenance.

Progress in our understanding of the molecular biology of estrogen action offers new opportunities to create designer estrogens for each target site. The diagram in Fig. 4 illustrates the possibilities, based on current knowledge, that could exist to interpret any ligand originally designated an "antiestrogen" to active estradiol-responsive genes. There are three potential research strategies. First, a ligand like tamoxifen may bind to the ER but different cells may have different associated proteins that help to form a transcription unit at an estrogen response element on the DNA. The estrogen-responsive gene could be turned on by tamoxifen in a target tissue if large amounts of the associated protein acted to enhance transcription of the imperfect receptor complex. A second mechanism is binding of the antiestrogen ER complex to an alternate site on the promoter region to override inhibitory responses and initiate gene transcription unilaterally. Although some evidence for the mechanism has been presented, the precise molecular events remain to be elucidated. Finally, a second ER, described as the β-receptor, has been discovered. The molecule has sequence homology with the classical ER (α) in the DNA-binding domain, but there is low homology in the ligand-binding domain. This opens the door for comparative structure-activity relationships with novel ligands once the tissue and cellular distribution of ERβ is established.

These fundamental advances in our basic knowledge, and the successful clinical application of antiestrogens to treat disease have encouraged a search for new agents for clinical use (Gradishar and Jordan 1997). At least a dozen major pharmaceutical companies have embarked upon programs of research and development, and numerous new agents will be introduced as medicines

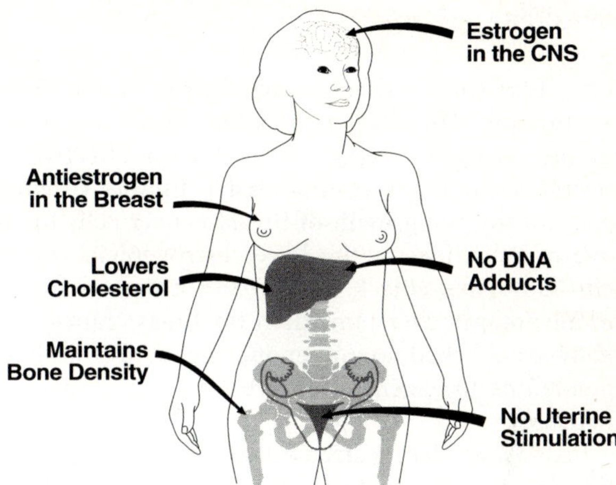

Fig. 3. The development of the ideal targeted antiestrogen to prevent the development of breast and endometrial cancer. The compound would act as a designer estrogen at important target sites for estrogen around a woman's body. As a result compounds could be used to prevent osteoporosis and coronary heart disease, but the beneficial side effect would be the prevention of breast and endometrial cancer

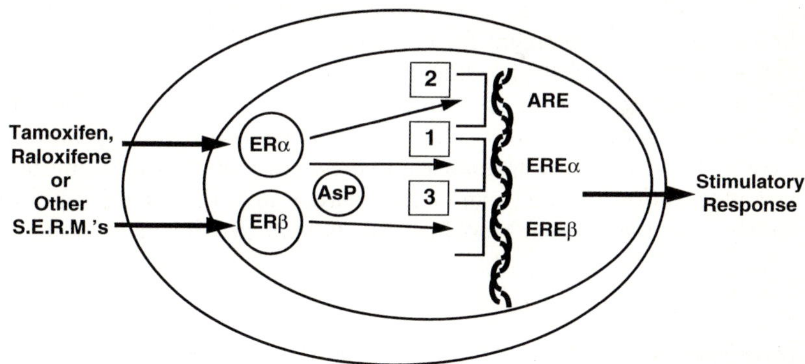

Fig. 4. The possible mechanism of action to explain the estrogen-like effects of the "nonsteroidal antiestrogens." There are three possible signal transduction pathways receiving attention. Firstly, the classic estrogen receptor (ERα) could bind the ligand but a tissue-specific excess of an associated proteins (*AsP*) would enable the complex to transcribe estrogen-responsive genes. Alternately, the complex could interact with an antiestrogen response element (*ARE*) rather than an estrogen response element (*ERE*) in the promoter region of a target gene. This interaction could have a dominant effect of encouraging promotion of gene transcription. Lastly, the discovery of a second receptors, *ERβ*, has raised the possibility that selective tissue distribution of the *ERβ* could account for tissue selectivity if a compound binds selectively to cause the activation of the complex

by the turn of the century. However, raloxifene, the compound initially found to prevent bone loss and mammary carcinogenesis in the laboratory, is now approved as a preventive for osteoporosis in postmenopausal women.

Raloxifene

Raloxifene (or keoxifene) started drug development as a potential breast cancer therapy. The drug is a potent antiestrogen with a high binding affinity for the estrogen receptor. Raloxifene is effective in controlling the growth of carcinogen-induced rat mammary tumors (Clemens et al. 1983), and analogues control the growth of breast cancer cells in culture. The potential advantage of raloxifene is the lower estrogenicity in the rodent uterus compared with tamoxifen (Black et al. 1983); however; in 1985 raloxifene demonstrated no advantages over tamoxifen for breast cancer treatment. Tamoxifen was already established as an endocrine adjuvant therapy and has been recommended as the agent of choice by a consensus panel of the National Cancer Institute.

In 1987 we demonstrated two important facts. Both raloxifene and tamoxifen would maintain bone density in rats, and both antiestrogens prevented rat mammary carcinogenesis (Jordan et al. 1987; Gottardis and Jordan 1987). We proposed a paradigm shift: develop targeted drugs for the prevention of osteoporosis and the prevention of breast and endometrial cancer could be a beneficial side effect. Our original findings have been confirmed and extended by others (Black et al. 1994; Sato et al. 1995) and, based on the laboratory profile (Fig. 5), raloxifene has now been evaluated in international clinical trials as a treatment for osteoporosis. At the same time raloxifene has been evaluated carefully for side effects. To date raloxifene shows little or no estrogen-like activity in the human uterus. All the pieces are being assembled to introduce a new concept to general medicine: a prevention maintenance therapy for the woman who wishes to embark on a long-term health care intervention. By the turn of the century new therapeutic options will be available for the woman who has risk factors for the major killers of post-

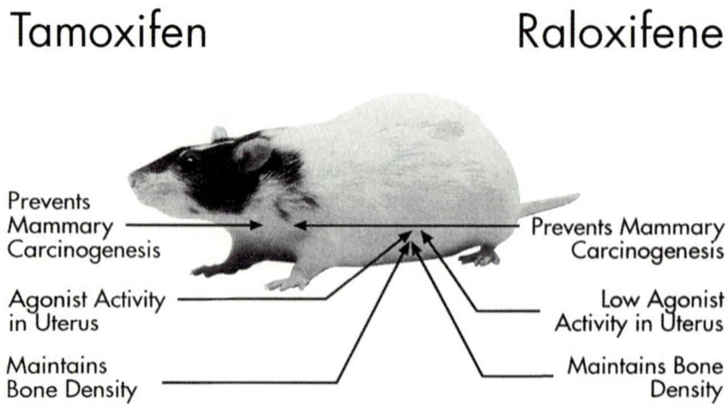

Fig. 5. The biological basis for the selection of raloxifene to be tested as a preventive for osteoporosis. The compound exhibits target site specificity bone density is maintained in ovariectomized rats and circulating cholesterol is reduced. At the same time raloxifene has virtually no estrogen-like effect on the uterus and prevents rat mammary carcinogenesis

menopausal women: osteoporosis, coronary heart disease, breast and endometrial cancer.

Acknowledgments. I am extremely grateful to the Lynn Sage Breast Cancer Foundation of Northwestern Memorial Hospital for their continuing support of our breast cancer program. Special thanks go to Henry Muenzner for preparing the figures.

References

Assikis VJ, Neven P, Jordan VC, Vergote I (1996) A realistic clinical perspective of tamoxifen and endometrial carcinogenesis. Eur J Cancer 32:1464–1476

Beatson GT (1896) On the treatment of inoperable cases of carcinoma of the mamma: suggestions for a new method of treatment with illustrative cases. Lancet II:104–107, 162–167

Black LJ, Jones CD, Falcone JF (1983) Antagonism of estrogen action with a new benzothiophene-derived antiestrogen. Life Sci 32:1031–1036

Black LJ, Sato M, Rowley ER, Magee DE, Bekele A, Williams DC, Cullinan GJ, Bendele R, Kauffman RF, Bensch WR (1994) Raloxifene (LY139481 HCI) prevents bone loss and reduces serum cholesterol without causing uterine hypertrophy in ovariectomized rats. J Clin Invest 93:63–69

Boyd S (1900) On oophorectomy in cancer of the breast. BMJ II:1161–1167

Breast Cancer Trials Committee, Scottish Trials Office (1987) Adjuvant tamoxifen in the management of operable breast cancer. Lancet II:171–175

Clemens JA, Bennett DR, Black LJ, Jones CD (1983) Effects of a new antiestrogen keoxifene (LY156758) on growth of carcinogen induced mammary tumors and on LH and prolactin levels. Life Sci 32:2869–2875

Cole MP, Jones CTA, Todd IDH (1971) A new antioestrogenic agent in late breast cancer. An early clinical appraisal of ICI 46474. Br J Cancer 25:270–275

Costantino JP, Kuller LH, Ives DG, Fisher B, Dignam J (1997) Coronary heart disease mortality and adjuvant tamoxifen therapy. J Natl Cancer Inst 89:776–782

Cuzick J, Baum M (1985) Tamoxifen and contralateral breast cancer. Lancet II:282

Early Breast Cancer Trialists' Collaborative Group (1992) Systemic treatment of early breast cancer by hormonal, cytotoxic or immune therapy. 133 randomized trials involving 31000 recurrences and 24000 deaths among 75000 women. Lancet 339:1–15, 71–85

Fisher B, Dignam J, Bryant J, DeCellis A, Wickerman DL, Wolmark N, Costantino JP, Redmond C, Fisher ER, Bowman DM, Deschenes L, Dimitrov NV, Margolese RG, Robidous A, Shibata H, Terz J, Paterson AH, Feldman MI, Farrar W, Evans J, Lickley HL (1996) Five years versus more than five years of tamoxifen therapy for breast cancer patients with negative lymph nodes and estrogen receptor-positive tumors. J Natl Cancer Inst 88:1529–1542

Fisher B, Costantino JP, Wickerhan DL, Redmond CK, Kovanah M, Cronin WM, Vogel V, Robidous A, Dimitrov NV, Arkins J, Daly M, Wieard S, Tan-Chiu E, Ford L, Wolmark N and other NSABP investigators (1998) Tamoxifen for prevention of breast cancer. Repeat of the national surgical adjuvant breast and bowel project P-I study. J Natl Cancer Inst 90:1371–1388

Fornander T, Rutqvist LE, Cedermark B, Glas U, Matteson A, Silfersvard C, Skoog L, Somell A, Theve T, Wilking N, Askergren J, Hjalmer MD (1989) Adjuvant tamoxifen in early breast cancer occurance of new primary cancers. Lancet I:117–120

Furr BJA, Jordan VC (1984) The pharmacology and clinical uses of tamoxifen. Pharmacol Ther 25:127–205

Gottardis MM, Jordan VC (1987) The antitumor actions of keoxifene (raloxifene) and tamoxifen in the N-nitrosomethylurea-induced rat mammary carcinoma model. Cancer Res 47:4020–4024

Gottardis MM, Robinson SP, Satyswaroop PG, Jordan VC (1988) Contrasting action of tamoxifen on endometrial and breast tumor growth in the athymic mouse. Cancer Res 48:812–816

Gradishar W, Jordan VC (1997) Clinical potential of new antiestrogens. J Clin Oncol 15:840–852

Hardel L (1988) Tamoxifen and risk factor for carcinoma of corpus uteri. Lancet II:563

Harper MJK, Walpole AL (1967a) Mode of action of ICI 46474 in preventing implantation in rats. J Endocrinol 37:82–92

Harper MJK, Walpole AL (1967b) A new derivative of triphenylethylene: effect on implantation and mode of action in rats. Reprod Fertil 13:101–119

Horwitz RI, Feinstein AR (1986) Estrogens and endometrial cancer: response to arguments and current status of an epidemiologic controversy. Am J Med 81:503–507

Jordan VC (1974) Antitumour activity of the antiestrogen ICI 46474 (tamoxifen) in the dimethylbenzanthracene (DMBA) induced rat mammary carcinoma model. J Steroid Biochem 5:354

Jordan VC (1976) Effect of tamoxifen (ICI 46474) on initiation and growth of DMBA-induced rat mammary carcinomas. Eur J Cancer 12:419–425

Jordan VC (1994) The development of tamoxifen. In: Jordan VC (ed) Long-term tamoxifen for breast cancer therapy. University of Wisconsin Press, Madison, pp 3–26

Jordan VC (1997a) Tamoxifen treatment for breast cancer: concept to gold standard. Oncology 11:7–13

Jordan VC (1997b) Tamoxifen: a guide for clinicians and patients. PRR, Huntington

Jordan VC (1997c) Tamoxifen: the herald of a new era of preventive therapeutics. J Natl Cancer Inst 89:747–749

Jordan VC, Phelps E, Lindgren JU (1987) Effects of anti-estrogen on bone in castrated and intact female rats. Breast Cancer Res Treat 10:31–38

Killackey MA, Hakes TB, Pierce VK (1985) Endometrial adenocarcinoma in breast cancer patients receiving antiestrogens. Cancer Treat Rep 69:237–238

Kristensen B, Ejlertsen B, Dalgaard P, Larsen L, Holmegaard SN, Transbol I, Mouridsen HT (1994) Tamoxifen and bone metabolism in postmenopausal, low risk breast cancer patients: a randomized study. J Clin Oncol 12:992–997

Lerner LJ, Jordan VC (1990) Development of antiestrogens and their use in breast cancer. Cancer Res 50:477–489

Love RR, Weibe DA, Newcomb PA, Cameron L, Leventhal H, Jordan VC, Feyzi J, DeMets DC (1991) Effects of tamoxifen on cardiovascular risk factors in postmenopausal women. Ann Intern Med 115:860–864

Love RR, Mazess RB, Barden HS, Epstein S, Newcomb PA, Jordan VC, Carbone PP, DeMets DL (1992) Effects of tamoxifen on bone mineral density in tamoxifen on bone mineral density in postmenopausal women with breast cancer. N Engl J Med 326:852–856

Madigan MP, Ziegler RG, Banichou J, Bryne C, Hoover RN (1995) Proportion of breast cancer cases in the United States explained by well established risk factors. J Natl Cancer Inst 87:1681–1685

Magriples U, Naftolin F, Schwartz PE, Carcagiu MD (1993) High-grade endometrial carcinoma in tamoxifen-treated breast cancer patients. J Clin Oncol 11:485–490

McDonald CC, Stewart HJ (1992) Fatal myocardial infarction in the Scottish tamoxifen trial. Br Med J 303:435–437

McDonald CC, Alexander FE, Whyte BW, Forrest AP, McDonald CC, Stewart HJ (1995) Cardiac and vascular morbidity in women receiving adjuvant tamoxifen for breast cancer in a randomized trial. Br Med J 311:977–980

Nolvadex Adjuvant Trial Organization (NATO) (1985) Controlled trial of tamoxifen as a single adjuvant agent in the management of early breast cancer. Lancet I:836–840

Peto R (1996) Five years of tamoxifen or more. J Natl Cancer Inst 88:1791

Powles TJ, Hardy JR, Ashley SE, Farrington GM, Cosgrove D, Davey JB, Dowsett M, McKinna JA, Nash AG, Sinnett HD, Tillyer CR, Treleaven JG (1989) A pilot trial to evaluate the acute toxicity and feasibility of tamoxifen for prevention of breast cancer. Br J Cancer 60:126–133

Powles TJ, Tillyer CP, Jones AL, Ashley SE, Treleavan J, Davey JB, McKinna JA (1990) Prevention of breast cancer with tamoxifen: an update on the Royal Marsden pilot program. Eur J Cancer 26:680–684

Powles TJ, Jones AL, Ashley SE, O'Brien ME, Tidy VA, Treleavan J, Cosgrove D, Nash AG, Sacks N, Baum M (1994) The Royal Marsden Hospital pilot tamoxifen chemoprevention trial. Breast Cancer Rest Treat 31:73–82

Powles TJ, Hickish T, Kanis JA, Tidy A, Ashley S (1996) Effect of tamoxifen on bone mineral density measured by dual-energy X-ray absorptiometry in healthy premenopausal and postmenopausal women. J Clin Oncol 14:78–84

Rutqvist LE, Mattson A (1993) Cardiac and thromboembolic morbidity among postmenopausal women with early-stage cancer in a randomized trial of adjuvant tamoxifen. J Natl Cancer Inst 85:1398–1406

Sato M, Kim J, Short LL, Szemenda CW, Bryant HU (1995) Longitudinal and cross-sectional analysis of raloxifene effects on tibiae from ovariectomized rats. J Pharmacol Exp Ther 272:1251–1259

Swedish Breast Cancer Cooperative Group (1996) Randomized trial of two versus five years of adjuvant tamoxifen for postmenopausal early stage breast cancer. J Natl Cancer Inst 88:1543–1549

Tonetti D, Jordan VC (1996) The development of targeted antiestrogens to prevent diseases in women. Mol Med Today 2:218–223

Vogel VG (1996) Assessing women's potential risk of developing breast cancer. Oncology 10:1451–1461

Ward HWC (1973) Antiestrogenic therapy for breast cancer. A trial of tamoxifen at two dose levels. BMJ I:13–15

Ward RL, Morgan G, Dalley D, Kelly PJ (1993) Tamoxifen reduces bone turnover and prevents lumbar spine and proximal femoral bone loss in early postmenopausal women. Bone Miner 22:87–94

IV. Clinical Cancer Chemoprevention

Chemoprevention of Human Cancer:
A Reasonable Strategy?

Frank L. Meyskens, Jr.

Chao Family Comprehensive Cancer Center, University of California, (Irvine), Orange, CA, 92668, USA

Abstract

The field of chemoprevention of cancer in humans is at a teenage level of maturity. There is anticipation and energy, and some promising results have come in, but it's unclear whether the entire enterprise is worth the effort. Reflecting on the status of the organism and where we are in its developmental history is therefore an important exercise at this time. Empirical and philosophical perspectives are offered for several key questions: Why prevent Cancer? What is the preclinical evidence that chemoprevention of cancer in humans should work? What is the clinical evidence that chemoprevention agents work? What is the clinical evidence that chemoprevention agent don't work? What is the status of ongoing randomized phase III/IV chemoprevention trials? The answers to each of these questions provide a part of the scaffold for a logical platform for the launching of the chemoprevention imperative as an integral part of our approach to the overall management of human cancer.

Why Prevent Human Cancer?

The best treatment of human cancer is its prevention. To which some have said 'You're only doing this "prevention stuff" until we can find a cure. Right?' Well, no. About 15 years ago this dialogue actually occurred, following a presentation I had made to the Southwest Oncology Group, a premiere cooperative therapeutics group in the United States. Indeed, if the treatment of a cancer were simple and without major consequences to the host then treatment might be enough, since in the phenomenon of risk a particular cancer in any one individual is uncommon and at least in nonhereditary associated malignancies (the majority of cancers) its appearance is not predictable – even though 50% of the population will develop a serious cancer in their lifetime and 30% of individuals in advanced societies will die of this disease.

Recent Results in Cancer Research, Vol. 151
Senn/Costa/Jordan (Eds.): Chemoprevention of Cancer
© Springer-Verlag Berlin · Heidelberg 1999

The conundrum, then, is that cancer overall is common in the population, but that any particular cancer in any one individual at any one point in time is relatively rare. This might suggest that only individuals at very high risk for cancer should enter prevention trials. However, progress in reducing morbidity and mortality from cardiovascular disease has been largely achieved by the broad application of preventative strategies – lowering of blood pressure and cholesterol levels. To date, though, a marker of risk for cancer equivalent to cholesterol level or blood pressure has not been correlated with the outcome of cancer or its chemoprevention, and consequently agents that are being tested in cancer chemoprevention trials must utilize changes in histologically identifiable preneoplasia or decreased cancer incidence for measurement of an effect. This approach has considerable drawbacks: definitive trials require large numbers of individuals on an intervention for a long period of time to be able to show a significant difference from an appropriate control group, and such investigations are very expensive to conduct. Another complicating factor is that candidate chemoprevention agents should have minimal to no toxicity and the separation of toxicity and effectiveness is a problem for all drugs, which has been quite limiting in the development of chemoprevention agents. To date, drugs with few side effects have been ineffective and effective drugs too toxic vis-à-vis risk-to-benefit ratio. Nevertheless, despite these myriad difficulties, prevention strategies should be vigorously pursued: the treatment of cancer is difficult at best. Advances in management of most serious malignancies has been incremental and the cost of treatment has accelerated markedly in the last decade as new and more expensive drugs and biologicals have been developed and entered into the general usage.

What Is the Preclinical Evidence Suggesting that Chemoprevention of Cancer in Humans Should Work?

The epidemiology and experimental work that underlies the enthusiasm of a preventative approach to cancer in humans is substantial. Epidemiological data strongly and consistently support a protective effect of dietary fruits and vegetables against a broad array of cancers (Willett and MacMahon 1984). Pinning down the exact constituent(s) has been much more difficult. Major dietary components that have been or are under study include macronutrients (fat, fiber) and micronutrients (e.g. β-carotene, calcium, vitamin A).

The results of the major chemoprevention trials are summarized below; to date the outcomes have not been uniformly positive (Tables 1, 2). The identification of a large number of chemicals from fruits and vegetables as candidate chemoprevention compounds, and in the future their systematic preclinical experimental development, should lead to earlier discontinuation of ineffective agents than has been the case to date. It is also anticipated that the

Table 1. Results of major randomized chemoprevention trials: positive trials (*BCC* basal cell carcinoma, *SCC* small cell carcinoma, *RA* retinoic acid)

Target	Agent	Finding	Reference
Actinic keratosis (AK)	Etretinate	Suppresses AK	Moriarity et al. (1982)
Xeroderma pigmentosum	13-*cis*-RA	Suppression of SCC	Kraemer et al. (1986)
Skin (low risk)	Retinol (low dose)	Decrease by 25% in SCC but not BCC	Moon et al. (1995)
Leukoplakia	13-*cis*-RA	Regression	Hong et al. (1986)
Head and neck	13-*cis*-RA	Suppression of second aerodigestive cancers	Hong et al. (1990)
Stage I lung (resected)	Retinol (high dose)	Decrease in second lung malignancies	Pastorino et al. (1993)
Hepatoma	Polyprenoic acid	Decrease in second hepatomas	Muto et al. (1996)
Cervical intraepithelial neoplasia (CIN)	*trans*-RA (topical)	Regression of CIN II but not CIN III	Meyskens et al. (1994a)
Head and neck	13-*cis*-RA	Suppression of second cancers	Hong et al. (1990)

Table 2. Results of major randomized chemoprevention trials: negative trials

Target organ	Agent	Finding	Reference
Skin (high risk)	Retinol; 13-*cis*-RA	No effect	Levine et al. (1997)
Skin (moderate risk)	β-Carotene	No effect	Greenberg et al. (1990)
Skin (low risk)	Selenium	No effect	Clark et al. (1996)
Lung (bronchial metaplasia)	13-*cis*-RA	No effect	Lee et al. (1994)
Lung (smokers)	β-Carotene, α-tocopherol	Increase in number of lung cancers	ATBC (1994)
Lung (smokers, asbestosis workers)	β-Carotene plus retinol (low dose)	Increase in number of lung cancers	Omenn et al. (1996a,b)
CIN	Folic acid	No effect	Butterworth et al. (1992)
CIN	Folic acid	No effect	Childers et al. (1995)
CIN	β-Carotene	No effect	Romney et al. (1997)
CIN	β-Carotene	No effect	Berman[a]

[a] Personal communication.

most promising agents will be identified before large phase III and IV trials are undertaken.

Experimental approaches using both in vitro and in vivo assessment of effects on the various stages of carcinogenesis and transformation markers have clearly shown that the natural history of tumor development can be altered, suppressed, and in some cases entirely prevented by the judicious use of inhibitors (Wattenberg 1985). Synthetic compounds, particularly the retinoids used at pharmacologic doses, have shown considerable effectiveness in preclinical animal models (Lippman et al. 1987). Based on promising early clinical results with vitamin A and vitamin A derivatives (retinoids), a large number of new derivatives have been synthesized. Although "proof of principle" of retinoids as effective chemoprevention agents in human cancer has been demonstrated, the doses required have produced significant toxicity and their use has not therefore been advocated for widespread use.

What is the Clinical Evidence Showing Chemoprevention Agents Work?

The results of reported randomized phase III and IV chemoprevention trials and a few other critical studies are summarized in Tables 1 and 2. Important ongoing phase III/IV studies are summarized in Table 3. Only three compounds have been tested in enough trials to warrant general statements about their efficacy or effectiveness against human cancer as preventative compounds. These include retinol (vitamin A), 13-*cis*-retinoid acid (Accutane, Isotretinoin) and β-carotene.

Retinol has been rigorously tested for a chemoprevention effect, in two settings: in patients at relatively low or high risk for skin cancer (Moon et al. 1995) and in patients with resected (for cure) stage I lung cancer (Pastorino et al. 1993). In the former study of skin cancer, in over 2000 patients at mild/moderate risk for skin cancer the incidence of squamous cell carcinoma was reduced by 25% by retinol, although there was no effect on the incidence of basal cell carcinoma. However, in a group of patients at high risk for skin cancer neither the same dose of vitamin A nor a low (10 mg) dose of 13-*cis*-retinoic acid affected the development of second cutaneous cancers (Levine et al. 1997). In the study of stage I lung cancer second lung malignancies were significantly reduced and an adjuvant effect also seen; a follow-up study is being done, and results should be reported in the near future (Hakama 1997). Additionally, supplementation with 50 000 IU vitamin A in patients with chronic myelogenous leukemia has increased the time to blast crisis and overall survival (Meyskens et al. 1995).

The most widely discussed chemoprevention trials have been those using 13-*cis*-retinoic acid. A number of clinical studies have shown that this synthetic retinoid can suppress oral leukoplakia (Hong et al. 1986; Lippman et al. 1993), inhibit the appearance of skin cancers in patients with xeroderma pigmentosa (Kraemer et al. 1986), and prevent the development of second primaries in patients with low-stage oral cancers resected for cure (Hong et al. 1990).

Table 3. Major ongoing randomized chemoprevention trials

Target organ	Agent	Location
Breast	Tamoxifen	NSABP
Colon (polyps)	Calcium	Dartmouth
Colon (polyps)	Fiber (wheat bran)	Arizona
Prostate	Proscar	SWOG
Lung	Vitamin A/acetylcysteine	EROTC

Other positive trials with other retinoids also have been reported: suppression of actinic keratoses with the retinoid etretinate (Moriarity et al. 1982), inhibition by polyprenoic acids (an acyclic retinoid) of second hepatomas in patients "cured" of hepatoma (Muto et al. 1996), and enhanced regression of moderate grade cervical intraepithelial neoplasia by topical β-*trans*-retinoic acid (vitamin A acid) (Meyskens et al. 1994).

What Is the Clinical Evidence to Show that Chemoprevention Agents Do Not Work?

Clearly, the most discouraging studies have been related to the carotinoid β-carotene. In randomized trials this compound, used at doses of 30–50 mg/day or every other day, has been found ineffective in decreasing the number of new incident cases of lung cancer in smokers (ATBC 1994; Omenn et al. 1996a, b), skin cancer in individuals with moderate actinic damage (Greenberg et al. 1990), and colon polyps in participants with prior polyps (Greenberg et al. 1994). Additionally, two randomized studies have shown that β-carotene did not alter the natural history of cervical intraepithelial neoplasia (Berman, personal communication; Romney et al. 1997), despite promising phase II results (Manetta et al. 1996). These sobering findings suggest that considerable caution needs to be exercised in the development of even such seemingly benign compounds as β-carotene, particularly since the usage of this compound emanated largely from the enthusiastic presentation of the epidemiological evidence (Peto et al. 1981) when little experimental evidence was available. The only trial in which β-carotene (as part of an antioxidant cocktail) may have shown benefit was in a large group of Linxian Chinese who were at high risk for upper gastrointestinal cancer but with normal esophageal evaluation (Blot et al. 1993). However, those individuals who already had esophageal dysplasia did not appear to be helped (Li et al. 1993). A number of other important trials also using supposed chemoprevention agents that showed no benefit have also been reported:
- 13-*cis*-Retinoic acid failed to alter the natural history of bronchial metaplasia (Lee et al. 1993), despite positive results in a much smaller trial in which etretinate was used (Gouveia et al. 1982).
- Supplemental folic acid was not effective in reversing cervical intraepithelial neoplasia (Butterworth et al. 1992; Childers et al. 1995).
- Selenium supplementation was not effective in preventing subsequent skin cancer in patients with actinic damage (Clark et al. 1996). Interestingly, the incidence of both prostate and colon cancer were decreased in this trial.

What Is the Status of Other Ongoing Randomized Phase III/IV Chemoprevention Trials?

There are several large studies for which accrual is complete or nearly so and follow-up is in progress (Table 3). Results can be anticipated in 1–3 years. These include:

- Calcium supplementation in patients with prior colon polyps. Both the epidemiological and the experimental data are strong and consistent, and I predict a lowering of polyp recurrence in the treatment arm.
- Wheat bran supplementation in patients with prior colon polyps. The epidemiological data are moderately strong and the experimental data, generally supportive. I predict that fiber will have a moderate, but nonsignificant, effect on polyp recurrence.
- Tamoxifen (an antiestrogen) in women at increased risk for breast cancer. The underlying experimental and available clinical data is impressive: tamoxifen should produce a 50% or greater decrease in breast cancer incidence.
- Proscar (an inhibitor of 5-OH reductase) in men at risk for prostate cancer. The underlying experimental rationale is only fair, and the agent is weak. I predict no effect of the agent on prostate cancer appearance.
- Vitamin A/acetylcysteine or a combination of both in patients with prior resected low-stage lung cancer. The experimental data are supportive (but complex) at the mechanistic level, but animal data is only so-so. However, clinical data are supportive of a vitamin A effect. I predict that vitamin A will reduce second malignancies but that the combination and acetycysteine alone will each be ineffective.

In addition to these trials systematic development has continued of several other compounds (Kelloff et al. 1996) for chemoprevention in humans, which have passed phase II testing and are ready for phase III/IV trials (Table 4). Most notably these include the polyamine synthesis inhibitor difluoromethylornithine (Meyskens et al. 1994b), the nontoxic retinoid 4-hydroxyphenylretinamide (Chiesa et al. 1992), and several nonsteroid anti-inflammatory agents, including aspirin, sulindac, and ibuprofen (Garewal 1992; Krishnan and Brenner 1996). Many other compounds are also being developed.

Table 4. Most notable compounds under development for chemoprevention

Agent	Biochemical effect	Target organs
DFMO	Polyamines	Colon, prostate, cervix
4HPR	Nuclear receptors	Breast
NSAID	Prostaglandin	Colon

Does Chemoprevention Work?

Although the results are mixed, on balance "proof of principle" has been shown in the clinical setting. The experience with chemoprevention of cancer to date highlights several issues that should allow for more rapid and directed development of these agents and consequently phase III trials that result in new advances. The major principles, I think, should include:

- Agents should not be selected on the basis of epidemiological results alone. Experimental data should be positive before a compound is advanced to the clinical setting.
- Compounds selected on the grounds of experimental approaches should be effective at low doses and/or exhibit low toxicity.
- Modulation of a relevant biochemical or biological marker in the tissue of relevance needs to be shown before the agent can be advanced in the clinical trials hierarchy (Meyskens 1991, 1992; Kelloff et al. 1996).
- Selection of drugs for the long (generally 12 months) phase IIb trials and subsequent phase III studies should be judicious (Goodman 1992).

My overall estimate is that the field of cancer chemoprevention is about a decade behind cardiovascular chemoprevention and in comparison to cancer treatment somewhere in the early 1960s. However, the slope in progress of cancer chemoprevention is likely to be steep, since many trials are nearing completion, progress in understanding cancer causation has been explosive in the last 15 years, and the study of the basic biology of risk (genetics), carcinogenesis, and progression of human precancers and cancers has become a major focus of scientists and clinicians in the last few years.

Acknowledgements. Supported in part from a grant from the NIH (P30CA62203). I thank Susan Scott for excellent administrative assistance in the preparation of this manuscript.

References

ATBC (1994) The effect of vitamin E and beta carotene on the incidence of lung cancer and other cancers in male smokers. The Alpha-Tocopherol, Beta Carotene Cancer Prevention Study Group. N Engl J Med 330:1029–1035

Benner SE, Pajoak TF, Lippman SE et al (1994) Prevention of second primary tumors with isotretinion in patients with squamous cell carcinoma of the head and neck: long term follow-up. J Natl Cancer Inst 86:140–141

Bertram JS, Kolonel LN, Meyskens FL Jr (1987) Rationale and strategies for chemoprevention of cancer in humans. Cancer Res 47:3012–3031

Blot WJ, Li J-Y, Taylor PR et al (1993) Nutrition intervention trials in Linxian, China: supplementation with specific vitamin/mineral combinations, cancer incidence, and disease-specific mortality in the general population. J Natl Cancer Inst 85:1483

Butterworth CE Jr, Hatch KD, Soung SJ et al (1992) Oral folic acid supplementation for cervical dysplasia: a clinical intervention trial. Am J Obstet Gynecol 166:803–809

Childers JM, Chu J, Voight L et al (1995) Chemoprevention of cervical cancer with folic acid: a phase III SWOG intergroup study. Cancer Epidemiol Biomarkers Prev 4:155–159

Chiesa F, Traditi N, Marazza M et al (1992) Prevention of local relapses and new localizations of oral leukoplakia with the synthetic retinoid fenretimide (4-HPR): preliminary results. Eur J Cancer 28:97–102

Clark LC, Combs GF Jr, Turnbull BW et al (1996) Effects of selenium supplementation for cancer prevention in patients with carcinoma of the skin. A randomized controlled trial. Nutritional Prevention of Cancer Study Group 276:1957–1963

Costa A, Formelli F, Chiesa F et al (1994) Prospects of chemoprevention of human cancers with the synthetic retinoid Fenretimide. Cancer Res 54:2032–2036 s

Garewal HS (1992) Aspirin in the prevention of colorectal cancer. Ann Intern Med 121:303–306

Goodman GE (1992) The clinical evaluation of cancer chemoprevention agents: defining and contrasting phase I, II, and III objectives. Cancer Res 52:2752–2758

Gouveia J, Mathé G, Heranand T et al (1982) Degree of bronchial metaplasia in heavy smokers and its regression after treatment with a retinoid. Lancet II:710–712

Greenberg ER, Baron JA, Stukel TA et al (1990) A clinical trial of beta carotene to prevent basal cell and squamous cell cancers of the skin. N Engl J Med 323:789–794

Greenberg ER, Baron JA, Tostenson TS et al (1994) A clinical trial of antioxidant vitamins to prevent colorectal adenoma. N Engl J Med 331:141–146

Hakama M (1997) Chemoprevention research in Europe. Int J Cancer 10:30–31

Hong WK, Endicott J, Intre LM et al (1986) 13-*cis*-Retinoic acid in the treatment of oral leukoplakia. N Eng J Med 315:1501–1505

Hong WK, Lippman SM, Itri LM et al (1990) Prevention of second primary tumors with isotretinoin in squamous cell carcinoma of the head and neck (SCCHN). N Engl J Med 323:795–801

Kelloff GJ, Crowell JA, Hawk ET et al (1996) Strategy and planning for chemopreventive drug development; clinical development phase II. J Cell Biochem Suppl 26:64–71

Kraemer KH, DiGiuvanna JJ, Moshell et al (1986) Prevention of skin cancer in xeroderma pigmentosium with the use of oral isotretinoin. N Engl J Med 318:1633–1637

Krishnan K, Brenner DE (1996) Chemoprevention of colorectal cancer. Gastroenterol Clin North Am 25:821–858

Lee JS, Lippman SM, Benner SE et al (1994) Randomized placebo-controlled trial of isotretinoin in chemoprevention trial of bronchial squamous metaplasia. J Clin Oncol 12:937–945

Levine NS, Moon TE, Cartmel B et al (1997) Randomized trial of retinol and 13-*cis*-retinoic acid for patients at high risk for skin cancer recurrence. Cancer Epidemiol Biomarkers Prev (in press)

Li JY, Taylor PR et al (1993) Nutrition intervention trials in Linxian, China: multivitamin/mineral supplementation, cancer incidence, and disease-specific mortality among adults with esopheal dysplasia. J Natl Cancer Inst 85:1482

Lippman S, Kolonel LN, Meyskens FL Jr (1987) Retinoids as preventive and therapeutic anticancer agents: I, II. Cancer Treat Rep 71:391–405, 493–515

Lippman SM, Batsakis JG, Toth BB et al (1993) Comparison of low dose isotretinoin with beta carotene to prevent oral carcinogenesis. N Eng J Med 328:12–20

Manetta A, Schubbert T, Chapman J et al (1996) β-Carotene treatment of cervical intraepithelial neoplasia: a phase II study. Cancer Epidemiol Biomarkers Prev 5:929–932

McClarty JW, Holiday DB, Giraud WM et al (1995) β-Carotene, vitamin A, and lung cancer chemoprevention: results of an intermediate endpoint study. Am J Clin Nutr 62:1431 S

Meyskens FL Jr (1991) Biology and intervention of the premalignant process. Cancer Bull 43:475–478

Meyskens FL Jr (1991) Biomarker intermediate endpoints and cancer prevention. Monogr Natl Cancer Inst 1992/13:177

Meyskens FL, Surwit ES, Moon TE et al (1994 a) Enhancement of regression of cervical intraepithelial neoplasia II (moderate dysplasia) with topically applied all-*trans* retinoic acid: a randomized trial. J Natl Cancer Inst 86:539–543

Meyskens FL, Emerson SS, Pelot D, Meshkinpour L et al (1994b) dose de-escalation chemoprevention trial diflouromethylornithine in patients with colon polyps. J Natl Cancer Inst 86:1122–1130

Meyskens FL Jr, Kopecky KJ, Appelbaum FR et al (1995) Effects of vitamin A on survival in patients with chronic myelogenous leukemia: a SWOG randomized trial. Leuk Res 19:605–612

Moon TE, Carmel B, Levine N et al for The Arizona Study Group (1995) Chemoprevention and etiology of non-melanoma skin cancers. Paper presented at the Seventeenth Annual Meeting of the American Society for Oncology, Tucson, 20–23 March 1995

Moriarty M, Dunn J, Darragh A et al (1982) Etretinate in treatment of actinic keratosis: a double blind crossover study. Lancet I:264–366

Muto Y, Moriwaki, Ninomiya M et al (1996) Prevention of second primary tumors by an acyclic retinoid, polyprenoic acid, in patients with hepatocellular carcinoma. N Engl J Med 334:1561–1567

Omenn GS, Gooodman GE, Thronquist MD et al (1996a) Effects of a combination of beta carotene and vitamin A on lung cancer and cardiovascular disease. N Engl J Med 3334:1150–1155

Omenn GS, Goodman GE, Thronquist MD et al. (1996b) Risk factors for lung cancer and for intervention effects in CARET, the beta carotene and retinol efficacy trial. J Natl Cancer Inst 88:21–30

Pastorino U, Infante M, Maioli M et al (1993) Adjuvant treatment of stage I lung cancer with high-dose vitamin A. J Clin Oncol 11:1216–1222

Peto R (1981) Can dietary β-carotene materially reduce human cancer rates? Nature 290:201–208

Romney SL, Ho GYF, Palan PR et al (1997) Effects of β-carotene and other factors on outcome of cervical dysplasia and human papillomavirus infection. Gynecol Oncol 65:483–492

Wattenberg LW (1985) Chemoprevention of cancer. Cancer Res 45:1–11

Willet WC, MacMahon B (1984) Diet and cancer – an overview: I, II. N Engl J Med 310:633–639, 697–702

Chemoprevention of Colorectal Cancer

J. Faivre and C. Bonithon-Kopp

Registre Bourguignon des Cancers Digestifs (INSERM CRI 9505),
Faculté de Médecine, 7 Boulevard Jeanne d'Arc, F-21033 Dijon Cedex, France

Abstract

Epidemiological studies have emphasised the major role of diet in the aetiology of large bowel cancer. Attempts to identify causative or protective factors in epidemiological and experimental studies have led to some discrepancies. The time has come to test the most important hypotheses within the framework of intervention studies. Among studies specifically devoted to colorectal carcinogenesis, eight have been completed and five are ongoing. They evaluate the effect of the intervention on adenoma recurrence and, in three studies, on adenoma growth. Five intervention trials considering cardiovascular diseases and different cancer sites will provide data on the effect of the intervention on colorectal cancer incidence. Vitamins and antioxidants, fibre or calcium supplementation, aspirin therapy and dietary modifications are evaluated. Most of the available data do not support the idea of a protective effect of vitamins and antioxidants against colorectal carcinogenesis. It is too early to draw any conclusions on the effects of fibre, calcium supplementation, aspirin therapy and dietary intervention. The results of ongoing studies will be available within 2 years. If one of the evaluated interventions proves efficient, the benefits of a simple, safe and inexpensive prophylaxis for a very common cancer will be clear.

Introduction

The most recent estimates of the worldwide incidence of colorectal cancer rank it third among the most frequent cancers, with about 560 700 new cases per year (Parkin et al. 1993). It is a major public health problem in all developed countries in Western Europe, North America and the South Sea Islands. Despite advances in diagnostic techniques and treatment, the 5-year survival rates remain poor and are estimated to be 30% in Europe (Berrino et al. 1995). There is little improvement with time. Strong evidence indicates that a high proportion of colorectal cancers arise in adenomas. These lesions could

Recent Results in Cancer Research, Vol. 151
Senn/Costa/Jordan (Eds.): Chemoprevention of Cancer
© Springer-Verlag Berlin · Heidelberg 1999

be a potential target for secondary prevention as well as for primary prevention. Several arguments lend credence to the notion that the adenoma–carcinoma sequence is a multistep progress. Cancer can be prevented by intervention either at the stage of adenoma growth or at that of transformation into carcinoma.

Many case-control studies, and some cohort studies, have provided substantial epidemiological evidence for the overwhelming role of diet in the occurrence of the disease (Potter et al. 1993). There is fairly consistent evidence concerning the effect of vegetables as a protective factor and of caloric intake as a risk factor. There is some evidence relating fat intake or protein intake to colorectal cancer, whereas fibre intake, calcium intake and antioxidant vitamins may be inversely related to colorectal cancer. However, analytical studies have yielded equivocal findings. The data available are not sufficient to serve as a basis for firm specific dietary advice, but they provide attractive hypotheses, which in turn suggest a rational basis for a preventive approach. Faced with this situation, it is important to test these hypotheses within the framework of intervention studies in order to evaluate the possibilities of primary prevention. The objective of this report is to review the design, along with the available results, of randomized colorectal cancer chemoprevention trials. Only studies with cancer or precancerous lesions (i.e. adenomas) as the main end-points are included here. Studies evaluating the effect of drugs are not considered.

Vitamins and Antioxidant Trials

In recent years, much attention has been paid to the potential advantages of antioxidant vitamins, including β-carotene, retinoids, vitamin C, and vitamin E, and of other micoronutrients, such as selenium, as chemopreventive agents for large bowel cancer. The main features of these trials are summarised in Table 1. Among the 15 chemopreventive studies with colorectal carcinogenesis as an end-point, 11 are at least partly concerned with the possible preventive effect of vitamins and/or antioxidants. The population involved is represented as follows: in 6 studies subjects who had previously had adenoma and who were polyp free at the time of recruitment; in 2 studies, individuals with familial adenomatous polyposis previously treated by total colectomy and ileorectal anastomosis (Bussey et al. 1982; De Cosse et al. 1989); and in 3 studies, volunteers included in large trials assessing the effects of micronutrients supplementation on cancer sites and cardiovascular diseases (ATBC Study Group 1994; Physician's Health Study cited in Hennekens et al. 1996; Hercberg et al. 1993). The effect of vitamin C alone was tested in 1 study (Bussey et al. 1982), the effect of β-carotene alone in 4 studies (Greenberg et al. 1994; MacLennan et al. 1991; ATBC Study 1994; Hennekens et al. 1996) and the effect of vitamin E alone in 1 study (ATBC Study 1994). Vitamin C and vitamin E were evaluated in 2 studies (De Cosse et al.

1989; Mc Keown-Eyssen et al. 1988), and various combinations of vitamins and of antioxidants in 4 studies (Roncucci et al. 1993; Hofstad et al. 1995; Bonelli et al. 1994; Hercberg et al. 1993). All these studies were double-blind randomized trials except for the Modena study (Roncucci et al. 1993), in which the reference group had no treatment. All the studies except 2 had a parallel design, meaning that the effect of one or several treatments was compared with the effect of the placebo. A 2×2 factorial design was used in 2 studies (Greenberg et al. 1994; MacLennan et al. 1991). The advantage of this design was that it allowed an estimation of the effect of the two combined treatments and that it gave more power to the study than a parallel scheme with the same number of patients.

The main end-point was adenoma recurrence in 5 studies (McKeown-Eyssen et al. 1988; Roncucci et al. 1993; Greenberg et al. 1994; MacLennan et al. 1995; Bonelli et al. 1994), variation in size of adenomas left in situ in 3 studies (Bussey et al. 1982; De Cosse et al. 1989; Hofstad et al. 1992), and colorectal cancer incidence in 3 studies (ATBC Study 1994; Hennekens et al. 1996; Hercberg et al. 1993). Most trials aimed at evaluating the effect of supplementation on adenoma recurrence or adenoma growth were small. The only large study was the one carried out within the National Polyp Study in the USA (Greenberg et al. 1994). Trials using adenoma recurrence or adenoma growth as the primary outcome have the advantage of being relatively small in size because a large number of events are expected during follow-up. For instance, the rate of patients with new adenomas is expected to be 30% at 3 years. However, whereas a relatively small sample size is sufficient to give the power needed to test the effectiveness of the intervention, some studies are obviously too small to provide any firm conclusion. In contrast, studies with invasive cancers as the main end-point require several tens of thousands of subjects.

The duration of the studies varies according to the main end-point. Trials that use adenoma recurrence or adenoma growth as the main end-point have the advantage of being relatively short in duration, ranging from 2 to 5 years (Table 1). Studies with colorectal cancer as the primary outcome require a longer follow-up period, generally at least 10 years.

The degree of compliance with the supplements is of importance. It was between 70% and 85% in most studies: 73% (Bussey et al. 1982), 79% (De Cosse et al. 1989), 75% (McKeown-Eyssen et al. 1988), 86% (Greenberg et al. 1994), 81% (Hofstad et al. 1995). It was only 45% in 1 study (Roncucci et al. 1993). Compliance with the final endoscopy was 73% in the St. Mark's Study, 79% in the New York Study, 78% in the Toronto Study, 87% in the National Polyp Study, 72% in the Australian Study, 87% in the Oslo Study and only 26% in the Modena Study.

The first chemopreventive study concerning colorectal cancer carcinogenesis was performed at St. Mark's Hospital, London, on patients treated for polyposis coli with the rectum left in place (Bussey et al. 1982). In the treatment group, there was a non-significant trend to a reduction in the number of rectal adenomas and in the adenoma area compared with the control

Table 1. Study designs, end-points and results of chemoprevention trials of vitamins and antioxidants in colorectal cancer carcinogenesis

Study	Subjects with	Intervention	No. of subjects	Duration	End-point results
Bussey et al. 1982, London	Familial polyposis	Vitamin C 2 g/day	49	15–24 months	No significant reduction in the number of rectal adenomas
De Cosse et al. 1989, New York	Familial polyposis	Viatmin C 4 /gd/day + vitamin E 400 mg/day	58	4 years	No effect on the number of rectal adenomas
McKeown-Eyssen et al. 1988, Toronto	Previous adenoma	Vitamin C 400 mg/day + vitamin E 400 mg/day	185	2 years	No effect on adenoma recurrence
Roncucci et al. 1993, Modena	Previous adenoma	Vitamin A 30 000 IU/day + vitamin E 70 mg /day	255	3 years	Significant reduction in adenoma recurrence
Greenberg et al. 1994, USA	Previous adenoma	β-Carotene 30 mg/day + vitamin C 1 g/day + vitamin E 400 mg/day	864	4 years	No effect on adenoma recurrence
Hofstad et al. 1995, Oslo	Previous adenoma	β-Carotene 15 mg/day + vitamin E 75 mg/day + vitamin C 150 mg/day + selenium 101 mg/day	116	3 years	No effect on adenoma growth or adenoma recurrence
MacLennan et al. 1996, Australia	Previous adenoma	β-Carotene 20 mg/day	378	4 years	No effect on adenoma recurrence
Bonelli et al. 1994, Genova	Previous adenoma	β-Carotene 15 mg/day + vitamin E 75 mg/day + vitamin C 150 mg/day + selenium 101 mg/day	279	5 years	Adenoma recurrence
ATBC 1994, Finland	Male smokers 50–69 years	β-Carotene 20 mg/day + vitamin E 50 mg/day	29 133	4–13 years	No effect on colorectal cancer incidence
Hennekens et al. 1996, USA	Medical doctors	β-Carotene 50 mg on alternate days	22 000	5 years	No effect on cancer incidence
SUVIMAX, France, 1993	Volunteers	β-Carotene 6000 mg/day + vitamin C 120 mg/day + vitamin E 15 mg/day + selenium 101 mg/day + zinc 20 mg/day	15 000	8 years	Cancer incidence, cardiovascular diseases

group (the reduction was significant at the 9 month follow-up, but disappeared over the next follow-up periods). A study with a similar design was performed in New York (De Cosse et al. 1989). There was no effect of vitamin E and vitamin C on the number of adenomas.

Of the 5 published studies that have tested the effect of antioxidant vitamins on adenoma recurrence, 4 are negative and 1 is still on-going (Bonelli et al. 1994). A Canadian study found no effect of supplemental vitamins C and E on the rate of recurrence of adenomas over a 2-year period (McKeown-Eyssen et al. 1988). In an American study there was no evidence that β-carotene or vitamin C and vitamin E reduced the risk of new adenomas (Greenberg et al. 1994). Neither diet treatment appeared to be effective in any of the subgroups studied defined according to sex, age, number of previous adenomas and serum level at entry or subtypes of adenoma identified at follow-up examinations (number of colorectal adenomas, size of the largest adenoma and location of the adenomas). In the Oslo study, no effect of a combination of β-carotene, vitamin E, vitamin C, selenium and calcium was found on the adenoma growth of an adenoma <1 cm in size that had not been extirpated (Hofstad et al. 1995). Moreover, there was no effect either from year to year or when the size of the left-in adenoma and/or the location of the adenoma, gender and cancer among first-degree relatives were taken into account. In the Australian study there was the suggestion of an adverse effect: the recurrence rate of large adenomas (>1 cm) increased (borderline significance) in the group receiving β-carotene supplementation. In contrast, a trial in Modena showed a significant reduction in the adenoma recurrence rate in patients receiving vitamins A, C and E compared with non-treated patients (Roncucci et al. 1993). The numbers of patients with a new adenoma at colonoscopy were 4 of 49 treated and 28 of 54 untreated patients. The main limitations of this study were the small number of patients (resulting in a lack of precision in efficacy estimates), the short follow-up period (only a quarter of the subjects had a colonoscopy after 2 years) and the fact that a substantial proportion of randomly assigned patients did not undergo a follow-up colonoscopy at all. Because of these limitations, the results of this study need to be regarded with caution.

Some results are also available from the large trials that have colorectal cancer incidence as an end-point. The Alpha Tocopherol, Beta Carotene, Lung Cancer Prevention Study in Finland was logistically a success (ATBC Study 1994). A total of 29133 male smokers aged 50–69 years participated in the chemoprevention trial, accumulating 169751 follow-up years. During the course of the study, 68 incident cases of colorectal cancer appeared in the α-tocopherol group versus 81 in the group not receiving α-tocopherol, and 76 in the β-carotene group versus 73 in the group and receiving β-carotene. In the United States, 22071 male physicians aged 40–84 years were randomized in a double-blind placebo-controlled trial of β-carotene, 50 mg on alternate days. Fewer than 1% had been lost to follow-up and compliance was 78% in the group that received β-carotene. Overall, 167 colorectal cancers were diagnosed in the intervention group and 174 in the placebo group (Hennekens et al. 1996).

The SUVIMAX study in France is still-going (Hercberg et al. 1993). No data on colorectal cancer incidence were reported from the CARET study (Ommen et al. 1996). A total of 18134 subjects at high risk of lung cancer (heavy smokers and asbestos-exposed workers) were included to assess the effect of β-carotene and vitamin A. This study was stopped prematurely because the active treatment group was found to have a significantly higher risk of lung cancer than the placebo group.

A lot of information is available on the effect of antioxidant vitamins on colorectal cancer carcinogenesis. This information allows the conclusion that antioxidant vitamins and micronutrients have no effect on adenoma recurrence, adenoma growth or colorectal cancer risk.

Fibre Trials

The results of analytical studies on dietary fibre are rather contradictory. It must be emphasised that dietary fibre is not a homogeneous entity and that different components may have different physiological effects. Food composition tables lack data on the different types of dietary fibre. In this context, studies examining the effect of a single source of fibre on experimental carcinogenesis in rodents are of interest. Pectin, cellulose, lignin, guargum, alfalfa, carrageen and cutin seem to have little effect (Faivre et al. 1991). However, a protective effect has been observed in most studies for wheat bran and mucilaginous substances (such as ispaghula husk), particularly during the promoting phase. The relevance of these data to human cancer must be evaluated in intervention studies.

Fibre supplementation is proposed in four chemopreventive studies (Table 2). The effect of wheat bran (22.5 g/day) together with vitamins C and E has been evaluated in patients with familial polyposis and with the rectum left in place (De Cosse et al. 1989). Its effect on adenoma recurrence was studied in the Australian study, with a dose of 25 g/day (McLennan et al. 1995), and in the Arizona study, with 13.5 g/day (Vargas and Alberts 1992). A multicenter European study performed within the European Cancer Prevention Organisation (ECP) has been assessing a mucilaginous substance in the form of ispa-

Table 2. Study designs, end-points and results of chemoprevention trials of fibre in colorectal cancer carcinogenesis

Study	Subjects with	Intervention	No. of subjects	Duration	End-point results
De Cosse et al. 1989, New York	Familial polyposis	Wheat bran 22.5 g/day + vitamin C 4 g/ day + vitamin E 400 mg/day	58	4 years	Nonsignificant reduction in the number of rectal adenomas
MacLennan et al. 1995, Australia	Previous adenoma	Wheat bran 11 g/day	378	4 years	Significant reduction in the number of adenomas >1 cm in the low-fat/ high-fibre group
Vargas and Alberts et al. 1992, Arizona	Previous adenoma	Wheat bran 13.5 g/day	1 400	5 years	Adenoma recurrence
Faivre et al. 1997, Europe	Previous adenoma	Ispaghula husk 3.8 g/day	656	3 years	Adenoma recurrence

ghula husk, 3.8 g/day (Faivre et al. 1997). This dose was that proposed by the manufacturer to obtain stool bulking. Most of the above-mentioned studies are larger than the chemopreventive trials of vitamins. Their duration varies between 3 and 5 years. The compliance rate for fibre intake was 79% in the New York study (De Cosse et al. 1989) and 74% in the Australian study (MacLennan et al. 1995), and is currently 77% in the ECP study (intermediate results on 564 subjects who ended the study before April 1997). Compliance with the final colonoscopy is of great importance for the interpretation of the results. It was 92% at 2 years and 72% at 4 years in the Australian study (McLennan et al. 1995). In the ECP study, intermediate results indicate that compliance with the 3 year colonoscopy was 89%.

The first fibre chemopreventive study was performed in patients treated for polyposis coli who had undergone total colectomy and ileorectal anastomosis and who were followed up at the Sloan-Kettering Institute in New York (De Cosse et al. 1989). The ratio between the initial number of adenomas and that at the follow-up examination was the main trial outcome. The intent-to-treat analysis suggested a limited effect of the treatment in the group receiving wheat bran, vitamin C and vitamin E compared with the groups receiving vitamins alone or a placebo. There were significant differences at 33 and 39 months only. When compliance was taken into account there was a stronger benefit in the combined fibre – vitamin group, particularly at the 2-year midpoint of the study.

In the Australian multicentre study there was no evidence that any intervention reduced the recurrence rate of adenomas at 2 or 4 years (McLennan et al. 1995), but a significant reduction in the incidence of large adenomas ($\geq$1 cm) was found in the low-fat diet group. The effect was observed when the low-fat diet was combined with wheat bran. This study suggests that a low-fat diet combined with wheat bran supplementation may reduce the risk of adenoma growth in patients with small adenomas.

The final results from the ECP study and from the Arizona study will be available soon.

In conclusion, the results available provide some evidence for an inhibition of adenoma growth through a high-fibre diet and/or a low-fat diet. The results of ongoing studies are expected to provide further arguments tu support these conclusions.

Calcium Trials

It has been hypothesised that a high intake of calcium may decrease the risk of colorectal cancer. Support for this hypothesis was obtained from a 19-year prospective study in the USA and from the fact that oral intake of calcium may induce a more quiescent equilibrium of epithelial cell proliferation in the colonic mucosa of subjects at high risk of colorectal cancer. However, such results have been reported in only half of the cell proliferation studies, and only one out of six case-control studies suggests a protective effect of high calcium intake.

Four intervention studies aimed at evaluating the possibility of primary prevention of colorectal cancer with calcium supplements have been carried out or are on-going (Table 3). All these studies are investigating subjects with a previous history of colorectal adenoma. As mentioned before, such trials have the advantage of being both relatively small in size and short in duration. In the ECP study, it was estimated with an assumed 30% recurrence rate at 3 years in the placebo group that 210 subjects per group are needed to detect a 15% difference between the tested group and the placebo group ($a = 0.05$; power $= 0.90$, two-tailed test). As for the polyp growth study, it can be estimated that there is an even higher proportion of patients with an increase in size of the unresected adenoma. In the ECP study, eligible patients had to have at least one adenoma over 5 mm in diameter or two adenomas. This gives more power to the study because such subjects have a higher recurrence rate than subjects with only a small adenoma. All these studies use adenoma recurrence as the primary outcome. The Oslo study has the additional feature that the effect of the intervention on the growth rate of an adenoma less than 1 cm in diameter left in situ in the large bowel is to be evaluated. None of the on-going studies has colorectal cancer as the main end-point.

The calcium being tested in the four studies is in the form of calcium carbonate or calcium gluconolactate various doses: 1.2 g/day (Baron et al. 1995), 1.5 g/day (Rooney et al. 1994), 1.6 g/day (with a mixture of antioxidants; Hofstad et al. 1995) and 2 g/day (Faivre et al. 1997). The study duration varies from one to another. It was 2 years in one study, 3 years in two studies and 4 years in one study (Table 3). In the Oslo and the Nottingham studies a control colonoscopy was performed yearly. In the two other studies control colonoscopy has been planned only for the end of the study.

The degree of compliance is an important factor in the success of the study, since the study power depends on both the sample size and the degree of compliance with the intervention. The compliance rate was 88% in the

Table 3. Study designs, end-points and results of chemoprevention trials of calcium in colorectal carcinogenesis

Study	Subjects with	Intervention	No of subjects	Duration	End-point results
Hofstad et al. 1995, Oslo	See Table 1				
Rooney et al. 1994, Nottingham	Previous adenoma	Calcium 1.5 g/day	79	2 years	No effect on adenoma, recurrence
Baron et al. 1995, USA	Previous adenoma	Calcium 1.2 g/day	930	4 years	Adenoma recurrence
Faivre et al. 1997, Europe	Previous adenoma	Calcium 1.0 g/day	656	3 years	Adenoma recurrence

Nottingham study (Rooney et al. 1991), 81% in the Oslo study (Hofstad et al. 1995) and 73% in the ECP study (intermediate results on 564 subjects who ended the study before April 1997). Compliance with the final colonoscopy examination was 88% in the Nottingham study, 87% in the Oslo study and 89% in the ECP study (intermediate results).

The two completed studies were small. In the Nottingham study no effect of calcium was found on adenoma recurrence after 2 years; the recurrence rate was 11% in both the calcium and the placebo groups (Rooney et al. 1994). In the Oslo study no effect on polyp growth was found, but there was a possible protective role of calcium and antioxidants against new adenoma formation. The two on-going studies – the ECP study and the American study – are larger. They will provide complementary information within 1 year.

It is not yet possible to draw firm conclusions on the effects of calcium supplementation in colorectal carcinogenesis, particularly on adenoma growth or adenoma recurrence. On-going studies are expected to provide further information.

Aspirin Trial

Several lines of evidence support the notion that aspirin and other monosteroid anti-inflammatory drugs may prevent large bowel cancers. Most case-control and cohort studies indicate a 30%–50% reduction in risk of colorectal cancer among regular users of aspirin. The results are consistent both for colon cancer and rectal cancer mortality or incidence and for adenoma occurrence. The results are not uniform, however, and a few studies found no benefit with aspirin use.

Only one chemoprevention study has investigated the effect of aspirin on occurrence of colorectal cancer (Gann et al. 1993). In this study, performed in male physicians in the USA, one aspirin tablet (325 mg) or a placebo was taken every other day. This study was stopped after 5 years because of evidence of protection against myocardial infarction. No protection by aspirin against colorectal tumours was seen. The relative risk was 1.15 for cancer and 0.86 for adenomas for subjects randomized to aspirin group. The relatively short duration of treatment can explain this result. Some data suggest that regular aspirin use for 10 years or longer is required for the inverse association to become apparent. Furthermore, cancers found soon after randomization were probably present when aspirin therapy began and would most likely not have been affected by aspirin use. There is little information regarding the optimal dose of aspirin. Benefits and risks have to be better defined. Because of the known toxicity of aspirin there is not a sufficient basis to recommend aspirin to the public for preventing colorectal cancer.

Conclusion

Altogether 15 chemopreventive studies (sometimes with several arms) have been performed to evaluate the possibilities of primary prevention of colorectal cancer: 8 in Europe, 6 in North America and 1 in Australia. Study populations are made up of subjects with previous adenomas or with remaining adenomas (i.e. intermediate steps in the natural history of the disease) or of volunteers included in large trials on cardiovascular diseases and/or other cancers in which colorectal cancer risk is one of the end-points. In addition to chemoprevention studies, 3 studies consider dietary interventions. Such studies are more difficult to implement and evaluate than are chemopreventive studies. The first study of this type was performed in Toronto (McKeown-Eyssen et al. 1994). In the intervention group, a low-fat diet (20% of energy from fat) and a high-fibre diet (50 g/day) was advised. After 12 months of counseling, fat consumption was 25% of energy in the intervention group and 33% in the control group, and fibre consumption was 35 g and 15 g, respectively. There was a nonsignificantly reduced risk of adenoma recurrence in women and an opposite risk in men. Thus, the issue of a gender-related effect on adenoma recurrence remains a definite question to be addressed in much larger studies. In the Australian study, as already mentioned, a low-fat diet (<25% of calories from fat) was proposed in one arm of the study (MacLennan et al. 1995). The National Polyp Study proposed a low-fat diet (<20% of total calories from fat), a high-fibre diet (at least 18 g/kcal of wheat bran) and fruit and vegetables (5–8 servings per day) in the intervention arm (Freedman and Schatzkin 1992). Overall, 2 094 subjects have been randomized in this study aimed at evaluating adenoma recurrence.

This review does not consider trials with only indirect end-points. In such studies, available results are suggestive of treatment efficacy in reducing colorectal cancer risk, though not decisive. These results are of interest within intervention studies, as they represent a unique opportunity for better understanding of the pathogenesis of colorectal carcinogenesis. Levels of cell proliferation in the intestinal mucosa have been evaluated in several studies (MacLennan et al. 1991; Faivre et al. 1997). Changes in the proliferation pattern have been correlated with the risk of colorectal tumours. It is worth evaluating the effect of the intervention on colonic cell proliferation. A detailed analysis of bile acids and related compounds is also planned in some chemopreventive studies (Hofstad et al. 1995; Faivre et al. 1997). Their involvement in colorectal carcinogenesis has been put forward, and the objective of the intervention is to decrease their toxic effects. In this context, it is important to document changes in their concentrations in faeces, for better definition of their role in the initial phases of colorectal carcinogenesis. Assessments of the underlying nutritional status before and after the intervention are important in the interpretation of the results. Diet needs to be estimated, with particular emphasis on the main hypotheses concerning colorectal cancer carcinogenesis.

It can be concluded that most available data do not support a protective effect of antioxidant vitamins (vitamin C, β-carotene, vitamin E, association of these vitamins) or micronutrients (selenium, zinc) on adenoma recurrence and growth and/or colorectal cancer risk. Results from small calcium chemo-preventive studies are difficult to interpret, and the same applies to the effect of dietary fibre. Although results are conflicting, there are some arguments in favour of a protective effect of dietary fibre and/or a low-fat diet on adenoma growth. The results of on-going preventive studies will provide further data on the effect of calcium and fibre on colorectal carcinogenesis. They will be available within 1 year.

Acknowledgments. This study, performed within the ECP colon group, was supported for its coordination by the Europe Against Cancer Programme, the Association Contre Le Cancer (Brussels), the Association Luxembourgeoise Contre le Cancer and the French Ministry of Health (PHRC). The calcium and its placebo were provided by the Sandoz France Company. The fibre and its placebo treatment were provided by Reckitt and Colman (UK).

References

Alpha-Tocopherol, Beta Carotene Cancer Prevention Study Group (1994) The effect of vitamin E and beta carotene on the incidence of lung cancer and other cancers in male smokers. N Engl J Med 330:1029–1035

Baron JA, Tosteson TD, Wargovich MJ (1995) Calcium supplementation and rectal mucosal proliferation: a randomized controlled trial. J Natl Cancer Inst 87:1303–1307

Berrino F, Sant M, Verdecchia A, Capocaccia R, Hakulinen T, Esteve J (1995) Survival of cancer patients in Europa. The EUROCARE study. (IARC scientific publications no. 132). IARC, Lyon

Bonelli L, Conio M, Picasso M, Massa P, Dodero M, Ravelli P, Missale G, Bruzzi P, Aste H (1994) Chemoprevention of metachronous adenomas of the large bowel: a double blind randomized trial of antioxidants (abstract), 3rd United European Gastroenterology Week, Oslo, abstract book, A 61

Bussey HJR, De Cosse JJ, Deschner EE, Eyers AA, Lesser ML, Morson BC, Ritchie SM, Thomas JPS, Wadsworth JA (1982) Randomized trial of ascorbic acid in polyposis coli cancer. Cancer 50:1434–1439

De Cosse JJ, Miller HH, Lesser ML (1989) Effect of wheat fiber and vitamin C and E on rectal polyps in patients with familial adenomatous polyposis. J Natl Cancer Inst 81:1290–1297

Faivre J, Wilpart M, Boutron MC (1991) Primary prevention of large bowel cancer. Recent Results Cancer Res 122:85–99

Faivre J, Couillault C, Kronborg O, Rath U, Giacosa A, De Oliveira H, Obrador T, O'Morain C, ECP Colon Group (1997) Chemoprevention of metachronous adenomas of the large bowel; design and interim results of a randomized trial of calcium and fibre. Eur J Cancer Prev 6:132–138

Freedman LS, Schatzkin A (1992) Sample size for studying intermediate end points within intervention trials or observational studies. Am J Epidemiol 136:1148–1159

Gann PH, Manson JE, Glynn RJ (1993) Low-dose aspirin and incidence of colorectal tumours in a randomized trial. J Natl Cancer Inst 85:1220–1224

Greenberg ER, Baron JA, Tosteson TD, Freeman DM, Beck GJ, Bond JH, Colacchio TA, Coller JA, Frankl HD, Haile RW, Mandel JS, Nierenberg DW, Rothstein R, Snover DC, Stevens MM, Summers RW, Van Stolk RU (1994) A clinical trial of antioxidant vitamins to prevent colorectal adenoma. N Engl J Med 331:141–147

Hennekens CH, Buring JF, Manson JE et al (1996) Lack of effect of long-term supplementation with beta carotene on the incidence of malignant neoplasms and cardiovascular disease. N Engl J Med 334:1145–1149

Hercberg S, Briancon S, Favier A (1993) Le projet SUVIMAX/100000 volontaires pour la recherche en nutrition dans le domaine de la prévention. Cah Nutr Diet 1:55–64

Hofstad B, Vatn M, Hoff G, Larsen S, Osnes M (1992) Growth of colorectal polyps: design of a prospective, randomized, placebo-controlled intervention study in patients with colorectal polyps. Eur J Cancer Prev 1:415–422

Hofstad B, Almenningen K, Vatn M, Norheim Andersen S, Owen RW, Larsen S, Osnes M (1995) Effect of calcium and antioxydants on growth of colorectal polyps (abstract). Gut 37:A 34

McKeown-Eyssen G, Holloway C, Jazmaji V, Bright-See E, Dion P, Bruce WR (1988) A randomized trial of vitamins C and E in the prevention of recurrence of colorectal polyps. Cancer Res 48:4701–4705

McKeown-Eyssen GE, Bright-See E, Bruce WR, Jazmaji V, Toronto Polyp Prevention Group (1994) A randomized trial of a low fat high fibre diet in the recurrence of colorectal polyps. J Clin Epidemiol 47:525–536

MacLennan R, Bain C, Macrae F, Gratten H, Battistutta D, Bokey EL, Chapuis P, Goulston K, Lambert J, Wahlquist H, Ward M (1991) Design and implementation of the Australian polyp prevention project. Front Gastrointest Res 18:60–73

MacLennan R, Macrae FA, Bain C, Battistutta D, Chapuis P, Gratten H (1995) Randomized trial of intake of fat, fiber and beta carotene to prevent colorectal adenomas. J Natl Cancer Inst 87:1760–1766

Ommen GS, Goodman GE, Thornquist MD et al (1996) Effects of a combination of beta-carotene and vitamin A on lung cancer and cardiovascular disease. N Engl J Med 334:1150–1155

Parkin DM, Pisani P, Ferlay J (1993) Estimates of the worldwide incidence of eighteen major cancers in 1985. Int J Cancer 54:94–606

Potter JD, Slattery ML, Bostick RM, Gapstur SM (1993) Colon cancer: a review of the epidemiology. Epidemiol Rev 15:499–545

Roncucci L, Di Donato P, Carati L, Ferrari A, Perini M, Bertoni G, Bedogni G, Paris B, Svanoni F, Girola M, Ponz de Léon M (1993) Antioxidant vitamines or lactulose for the prevention of the recurrence of colorectal adenomas. Dis Colon Rectum 36:227–234

Rooney PS, Gifford KA, Clarke PA, Hardcastle JD, Armitage NC (1994) A double-blind randomized controlled of dietary calcium supplementation in individuals with adenomas (one-year results) (abstract). Dis Colon Rectum 37:P 41

Vargas PA, Alberts DS (1992) Primary prevention of colorectal cancer through dietary modification. Cancer 70:1229–1235

Computer to plate: Mercedes Druck, Berlin
Binding: Buchbinderei Lüderitz & Bauer, Berlin